Lyme Disease and The Nervous System

Louis Reik, Jr., M.D.

Associate Professor of Neurology
University of Connecticut Health Center
Farmington, Connecticut

1991
Thieme Medical Publishers, Inc. NEW YORK
Georg Thieme Verlag STUTTGART • NEW YORK

Thieme Medical Publishers, Inc.
381 Park Avenue South
New York, New York 10016

LYME DISEASE AND THE NERVOUS SYSTEM
Louis Reik, Jr., M.D.

Library of Congress Cataloging-in-Publication Data

Reik, Louis,
    Lyme disease and the nervous system / Louis Reik, Jr.
      p.   cm.
    Includes bibliographical references and index.
    ISBN 0-86577-394-7 (Thieme Medical Publishers).—ISBN
3-13-771701-9 (Georg Thieme Verlag)
      1. Lyme disease.   2. Nervous system—Infections.   3. Neurologic
manifestations of general diseases.   I. Title.
      [DNLM: 1. Lyme Disease.   2. Nervous System—pathology.   WC 406
R361L]
    RC155.5.R45   1991
    616.9'2—dc20
    DNLM/DLC
    for Library of Congress   91-800
                                                                              CIP

Important note: Medicine is an ever-changing science. Research and clinical experience are continually broadening our knowledge, in particular our knowledge of proper treatment and drug therapy. Insofar as this book mentions any dosage or applications, readers may rest assured that the authors, editors, and publishers have made every effort to ensure that such references are strictly in accordance with the state of knowledge at the time of production of the book. Nevertheless, every user is requested to carefully examine the manufacturers' leaflets accompanying each drug to check on his own responsibility whether the dosage schedules recommended therein or the contraindications stated by the manufacturers differ from the statements made in the present book. Such examination is particularly important with drugs that are either rarely used or have been newly released on the market.

Some of the product names, patents, and registered designs referred to in this book are in fact registered trademarks or proprietary names even though specific reference to this fact is not always made in the text. Therefore, the appearance of a name without designation as proprietary is not to be construed as a representation by the publisher that it is in the public domain.

Printed in the United States of America.

5 4 3 2 1

TMP ISBN 0-86577-394-7
GTV ISBN 3-13-771701-9

Contents

Preface

When, as a house officer at Yale in 1977, I first saw patients with nervous system Lyme disease, I thought it was a fascinating disease but assumed that it was of only regional importance. The events of the past 13 years have shown me how wrong I was. Lyme disease has proved to be widespread and common both here in the United States and worldwide. I have watched with interest as it has received increasing publicity, some of it the source of misconception, and have seen in my referral practice how it has become an increasing cause for concern among patients and their physicians. Yet many physicians remain relatively unsophisticated about Lyme disease, particularly about its neurologic manifestations, even in my home state of Connecticut where it was described first. I believe that this is true in part because there is no good single source for the neurologist to learn about the illness.

The purpose of this book is to fill this gap and provide an overview of how Lyme disease affects the nervous system. *Lyme Disease and the Nervous System* is a book for neurologists about the neurologic manifestations of Lyme disease. While it may be of interest also to neurosurgeons, internists, and pediatricians interested in infections of the nervous system, it is not meant to be an exhaustive review of the entire topic of Lyme disease. The epidemiology, etiology, pathology, pathogenesis, and general and laboratory features of Lyme disease are reviewed only in sufficient detail to allow the neurologist to understand the neurologic features of the illness in context and to allow their diagnosis on clinical grounds. The focus of this book is on the neurologic manifestations of the disease and their diagnosis and treatment.

When I set out to write this book, I did not really appreciate how much had been written about nervous system Lyme disease in the last 10 years, even though I remained interested in and continued to see patients with the disease since my first encounters with it. I am sure that, inevitably, I have neglected to include some important references. I am also sure that some of what I have written will be out of date by the time the book is published. I hope that I have been able to give an accurate view of the present state of our knowledge about this fascinating nervous system infection, nevertheless.

One additional explanation is necessary. Throughout the book I have referred to this borrelial infection as Lyme disease rather than Lyme borreliosis, which many now prefer. I find Lyme disease more euphonious and see no real reason to change it just because we know now that it is caused by *Borrelia burgdorferi*.

Louis Reik, Jr., MD
Farmington, Connecticut

Acknowledgments

I am indebted to many people whose help allowed me to write this book. Drs. Paul Duray, John Halperin, Alan MacDonald, Eugene May, Tom Schwan, Alan Steere, and Arnold Witte and Ms. Marge Anderson of Pfizer Central Research all generously allowed me to reproduce original material. Drs. Jim Donaldson and Tony Voytovich critically read portions of the manuscript, as did my wife, Dr. Hester Reik. Tony Voytovich also introduced me to the world of computers and helped me in my early attempts at learning to use one. The patient folks at Biomedical Communication at the University of Connecticut Health Center cheerfully reproduced the illustrations repeatedly whenever I changed my mind about how I wanted them to look (as I did often). Most importantly, my wife and children were enthusiastic and supportive throughout the whole venture, never complaining about the time I spent locked up with my word processor.

1

Introduction

Lyme disease, also called Lyme borreliosis, is a widely distributed multi-system disease caused by a tick-transmitted spirochete, *Borrelia burgdorferi*. Although symptoms of this infection were described first in Europe over a hundred years ago, the full clinical picture and worldwide distribution of Lyme disease have been recognized largely because of research in the last two decades. As a result of this research, Lyme disease is now known to be the cause of a wide range of treatable neurologic abnormalities.

The modern era in the understanding of Lyme disease began in 1975 when rheumatologists at Yale University learned from two parents of children who had arthritis of an epidemic of arthritis in the small town of Lyme, Connecticut, and established a surveillance system there and in two neighboring towns to identify children with inflammatory joint disease.[1,2]

They found 39 children and 12 adults who had developed a remitting, relapsing oligoarticular arthritis between 1972 and 1976. Epidemiologic evidence suggested that this arthritis was infectious and transmitted by an arthropod, as those affected lived in sparsely settled, forested parts of the towns; their symptoms usually began in summer or fall; and when more than one family member was affected, they often had the onset of symptoms in different years.[3]

The Yale investigators also discovered that 13 of the 51 had had an unusual rash before the arthritis started.[3] The rash began as a red papule and expanded centrifugally to form a ring with partial central clearing and resembled erythema migrans (EM), a skin lesion that was little known in the United States but common in Europe where it had been reported first in 1909.[4] European EM was known to be transmitted by an arthropod, the sheep tick, *Ixodes ricinus*, and to be infectious in nature—it had been transmitted from human to human by inoculation of material from the edge of the lesion[5,6]—but the nature of the infectious agent was not known. Lennhoff reported seeing spirochetes in mercury-stained sections of EM in 1948,[7] and

1

both Hollström[8,9] and Hellerström[10] successfully treated the lesion with penicillin; but when subsequent studies failed to confirm Lennhoff's findings, other agents were suspected, particularly viruses and rickettsiae.[11]

European EM appeared, moreover, to be related to two other tick-transmitted, antibiotic-responsive skin lesions, lymphocytoma cutis (LC) and acrodermatitis chronica atrophicans (ACA). The status of LC, a solitary skin lesion with lymphoid follicles resembling a lymph node, was remarkably similar to that of EM. LC was described first in 1911 by Burckhardt,[12] and had been linked to tick bites and known to occur together with EM as early as 1920.[13] Lennhoff had seen spirochetes in mercury-stained sections of lymphocytoma in 1948,[7] just as he had in EM, and Bianchi had established the beneficial effect of penicillin in 1950.[14] Moreover, the infectious nature of LC had been proved by Paschoud in 1957 and 1958 through human-to-human transmission experiments.[15]

The status of ACA, a chronic skin lesion characterized by acral swelling and discoloration followed by skin atrophy, was also similar to that of EM. ACA had been reported from Europe in the late 1800s,[16] but it was first named and characterized in detail in Herxheimer and Hartmann in 1902.[17] An infectious etiology was suspected early on, and spirochetes were implicated by reports of positive pallida reactions in patients with the lesion.[18] ACA had been treated successfully with penicillin,[19] and it was transmitted from human to human by implantation of skin biopsy specimens.[20] In addition, ACA in Europe was linked to tick bites, its distribution paralleling that of *I. ricinus*, and it was found to follow or accompany both EM and LC.[21]

European EM was also known to be followed by neurologic disease, an association that was already the subject of a rich European literature. The association was first noted in 1922 by Garin and Bujadoux,[22] who reported the case of a 58-year-old French farmer who developed neuralgic pains, paralysis of the deltoid muscle, meningoencephalitis, and spreading erythema after a tick bite. Other reports followed of patients with chronic meningitis after EM.[8,10,23] Then Bannwarth described 19 patients with tick bites followed by radicular pain, often in the dermatomal segment of the preceding bite, and chronic meningitis sometimes accompanied by peripheral and cranial nerve palsies, most commonly facial palsy.[24,25] Only two of his patients had EM, however. Subsequent reports by Schaltenbrand[26–28] and Bammer and Schenk[29] confirmed the relationship between EM, chronic meningitis, and painful peripheral neuritis and enlarged the neurologic spectrum of the illness to include myelitis and optic neuritis. The most detailed account of this illness, however, was given by Hörstrup and Ackermann[30] who named it tick-borne meningopolyneuritis (Garin-Bujadoux, Bannwarth). They described 47 patients, 9 of whom had had a tick bite and 15 of whom had EM, who developed neurologic disease during the summer months, characterized by radicular pains, lymphocytic meningitis, and peripheral and cranial neuritis. Meanwhile, other reports had linked lymphocytoma with polyradiculitis and pleocytosis[31] and acrodermatitis with peripheral neuropathy.[32]

But neurologic abnormalities had not been reported by the Connecticut patients, and European EM had not been associated with arthritis. When cultures and serologic tests done on their patients did not indicate infection with agents known to cause arthritis, the Yale investigators believed that they were reporting a new disease and named it "Lyme arthritis."[3]

The next year, the investigators identified 24 patients who developed the skin lesion, followed them prospectively, and confirmed the identity of the lesion as EM.[33] EM developed between May and August in all but one patient and followed an antecedent tick bite at the same site in three. Moreover, the lesion was followed by arthritis in many, and some patients also developed cardiac conduction defects or, like their European counterparts with meningopolyneuritis, lymphocytic meningitis and cranial or peripheral neuritis.

With their surveillance system in place, the Yale physicians continued to follow new patients prospectively and identified additional patients with the skin lesion, arthritis, or both in 1977.[34] Nine of 43 new patients recalled a tick bite at the site of EM. The responsible tick, saved by one of its victims, was identified first as *Ixodes scapularis* and then *Ixodes dammini*, a new species,[35] and field studies of the vector indicated that its geographic distribution paralleled that of the illness.[36]

Further prospective studies by the same investigators detailed the neurologic[37] and cardiac manifestations[38] of the disease and confirmed that North American EM, like the European form, responded to antibiotics.[39] Recognizing the multisystem nature of the illness, they renamed it "Lyme disease."[37] At the same time, increasing numbers of cases reported from outside Connecticut revealed the widespread distribution of the new illness in North America.[40]

But the identity of the infectious agent of Lyme disease eluded the Yale investigators. It was discovered instead by Dr. Willy Burgdorfer of the Rocky Mountain Laboratories in Hamilton, Montana.[41] Dr. Burgdorfer was searching for the vector of Rocky Mountain spotted fever on Long Island, New York, but was unable to find rickettsia in *Dermacentor variabilis*, the usual vector, so he began looking for them in *I. dammini*. He found spirochetes instead.

Familiar with the earlier European literature, Dr. Burgdorfer realized he might have discovered the agent of EM and Lyme disease and enlisted the help of Dr. Alan Barbour, his colleague at the Rocky Mountain Laboratory, in culturing the organism.[11] Dr. Barbour succeeded, and his success permitted them to demonstrate immunologically the relationship of the cultured spirochete to the agent of Lyme disease[41,42] and to show that inoculations of the cultured spirochete produced a similar disease in laboratory animals.[41] Finally, with Dr. Barbour's cultural techniques, the *I. dammini* spirochete was isolated from the blood, skin lesions, and cerebrospinal fluid (CSF) of patients with Lyme disease, proving its spirochetal etiology.[43,44]

The pace of discovery then accelerated. Within a year, similar spirochetes were isolated from ixodid tick vectors from both the western United States[45] and Europe,[46] demonstrated histologically in biopsied EM lesions,[47] and cultured from European patients with EM[48] and with meningopolyneuritis.[49,50] Shortly thereafter, the organisms were also demonstrated histologically in[51] and isolated from the skin lesions of patients with lymphocytoma[52] and acrodermatitis.[53] Determined to be a new species of *Borrelia*, the spirochete was named *Borrelia burgdorferi* in honor of its discoverer.[54]

The ability to grow *B. burgdorferi* in pure culture facilitated the laboratory exploration of both the organism's biology and its role in the pathogenesis of Lyme disease. It facilitated also the development of sensitive serologic tests that advanced the study of the epidemiology and natural history of Lyme disease and allowed the diagnosis of Lyme disease to be made on laboratory as well as clinical grounds.

As a result, our view of the spectrum of illness caused by *B. burgdorferi* infection, particularly the neurologic abnormalities, expanded further. Cases of isolated neurologic involvement without antecedent EM or subsequent arthritis were diagnosed serologically[55]; the occurrence of more severe central nervous system abnormalities in early Lyme disease was documented[56]; and previously unrecognized syndromes of chronic progressive borrelial encephalomyelitis,[57] polyneuropathy,[58] and encephalopathy[59] occurring in late Lyme disease were described for the first time.

Finally, recognition of the spirochetal etiology of Lyme disease and the ability to cultivate *B. burgdorferi* and test its antibiotic sensitivity *in vitro* led to the development of more effective antibiotic treatments for both the early manifestations of Lyme disease and its later neurologic and arthritic complications.[60–62]

References

1. Steere AC, Hardin JA, Malawista SE. Lyme arthritis: A new clinical entity. *Hosp Pract* 1978;13(4):143–158.
2. Steere AC, Malawista SE, Bartenhagen NH, et al. The clinical spectrum and treatment of Lyme disease. *Yale J Biol Med* 1984;57:453–461.
3. Steere AC, Malawista SE, Snydman DR. Lyme arthritis: An epidemic of oligoarticular arthritis in children and adults in three Connecticut communities. *Arthritis Rheum* 1977;20:7–17.
4. Afzelius A. Erythema chronicum migrans. *Acta Derm Venereol (Stockh)* 1921;2:120–125.
5. Binder E, Doepfmer R, Hornstein O. Experimentelle Übertragung des Erythema chronicum migrans von Mensch zu Mensch. *Hautarzt* 1955;6:494–496.
6. Sonck CE. Erythema chronicum migrans with multiple lesions. *Acta Derm Venereol (Stockh)* 1965;45:34–36.
7. Lennhoff C. Spirochaetes in aetiologically obscure diseases. *Acta Derm Venereol (Stockh)* 1948;8:295–324.
8. Hollström E: Successful treatment of erythema chronicum migrans Afzelius. *Acta Derm Venereol (Stockh)* 1951;31:235–243.
9. Hollström E. Penicillin treatment of erythema chronicum migrans Afzelius. *Acta Derm Venereol (Stockh)* 1958;38:285–289.
10. Hellerström S. Erythema chronicum migrans Afzelius with meningitis. *Acta Derm Venereol (Stockh)* 1951;31:227–234.
11. Burgdorfer W. Discovery of the Lyme disease spirochete and its relation to tick vectors. *Yale J Biol Med* 1984;57:515–520.

12. Burckhardt JL. Cited by Weber K, Schierz G, Wilske B, Preac-Mursic V. European erythema migrans disease and related disorders. *Yale J Biol Med* 1984;57:463–471.
13. Strandberg J. Regarding an unusual form of migratory erythema caused by tick bites. *Acta Derm Venereol (Stockh)* 1920;1:422–427.
14. Bianchi GE. Die Penicillinbehandlung der Lymphozytome. *Dermatologica* 1950;100:270–273.
15. Paschoud JM. Die Lymphadenosis benigna cutis als übertragbare Infektionskrankheit, IV: Mitteilung. *Hautarzt* 1958;9:311–315.
16. Buchwald A. Cited by Weber K, Schierz G, Wilske B, Preac-Mursic V. European erythema migrans disease and related disorders. *Yale J Biol Med* 1984;57:463–471.
17. Herxheimer K, Hartmann K. Über Acrodermatitis chronica atrophicans. *Arch Dermatol Syph* 1902;61:57–76.
18. Grüneberg T. Auffällige serologische Befunde bei Acrodermatitis chronica atrophicans Herxheimer. *Klin Wochenschr* 1954;32:935–936.
19. Thyresson N. The penicillin treatment of acrodermatitis atrophicans chronica (Herxheimer). *Acta Derm Venereol (Stockh)* 1949;29:572–621.
20. Götz H. Die Acrodermatitis chronica atrophicans Herxheimer als Infektionskrankheit. *Hautarzt* 1955;6:249–252.
21. Hauser, W. Zur Kenntnis der Akrodermatitis chronica atrophicans. *Arch Dermatol Syph* 1955;199:350–393.
22. Garin C, Bujadoux C. Paralysie par les Tiques. *J Med Lyon* 1922;71:765–767.
23. Lecinsky CG. Case of erythema chronicum migrans with meningitis. *Acta Derm Venereol (Stockh)* 1951;31:464–467.
24. Bannwarth A. Chronische lymphozytäre Meningitis, entzündliche Polyneuritis und Rheumatismus. *Arch Psychiatr Nervenkr* 1941;113:284–376.
25. Bannwarth A. Zur Klinik und Pathogenese der "chronischen lymphozytären Meningitis." *Arch Psychiatr Nervenkr* 1944;117:161–185.
26. Schaltenbrand G. Radiculomyelomeningitis nach Zeckenbiss. *Munch Med Wochenschr* 1962;104:829–834.
27. Schaltenbrand G. Durch Arthropoden übertragene Infektionen der Haut und des Nervensystems. *Munch Med Wochenschr* 1966;108:1557–1562.
28. Schaltenbrand G. Durch Arthropoden übertragene Erkrankungen der Haut und des Nervensystems. *Verh Dtsch Ges Inn Med* 1966;72:975–1005.
29. Bammer H, Schenk K. Meningo-Myelo-Radiculitis nach Zeckenbiss mit Erythem. *Dtsch Z Nervenheilk* 1965;187:25–34.
30. Hörstrup P, Ackermann R. Durch Zecken übertragene Meningopolyneuritis (Garin-Bujadoux, Bannwarth). *Fortschr Neurol Psychiatr* 1973;41:583–606.
31. Paschoud JM. Lymphocytom nach Zeckenbiss. *Dermatologica* 1954;108:435–437.
32. Hopf HC. Peripheral neuropathy in acrodermatitis chronica atrophicans (Herxheimer). *J Neurol Neurosurg Psychiatry* 1975;38:452–458.
33. Steere AC, Malawista SE, Hardin JA, Ruddy S, Askenase PW, Andiman WA. Erythema chronicum migrans and Lyme arthritis: The enlarging clinical spectrum. *Ann Intern Med* 1977;86:685–698.
34. Steere AC, Broderick TF, Malawista SE. Erythema chronicum migrans and Lyme arthritis: Epidemiologic evidence for a tick vector. *Am J Epidemiol* 1978;108:312–321.
35. Spielman A, Clifford CM, Piesman J, Corwin MD. Human babesiosis on Nantucket Island, USA: Description of the vector, *Ixodes (Ixodes) dammini*, n. sp. (Acarina: Ixodidae). *J Med Entomol* 1979;15:218–234.
36. Wallis RC, Brown SE, Kloter KO, Main AJ. Erythema migrans and Lyme arthritis: Field study of ticks. *Am J Epidemiol* 1978;108:322–327.
37. Reik L, Steere AC, Bartenhagen NH, Shope RE, Malawista SE. Neurologic abnormalities of Lyme disease. *Medicine (Baltimore)* 1979;58:281–294.
38. Steere AC, Batsford WP, Weinberg M, et al. Lyme carditis: Cardiac abnormalities of Lyme disease. *Ann Intern Med* 1980;93:8–16.
39. Steere AC, Malawista SE, Newman JH, Spieler PN, Bartenhagen NH. Antibiotic therapy in Lyme disease. *Ann Intern Med* 1980;93:1–8.
40. Steere AC, Malawista SE. Cases of Lyme disease in the United States: Locations correlated with distribution of *Ixodes dammini*. *Ann Intern Med* 1979;91:730–733.
41. Burgdorfer W, Barbour AG, Hayes SF, Benach JL, Grunwaldt E, Davis JP. Lyme disease—a tick-borne spirochetosis? *Science* 1982;216:1317–1319.

42. Burgdorfer W, Barbour AG, Hayes SF, Peter O, Aeschlimann A. Erythema chronicum migrans—a tickborne spirochetosis. *Acta Trop (Basel)* 1983;40:79–83.
43. Steere AC, Grodzicki RL, Kornblatt AN, et al. The spirochetal etiology of Lyme disease. *N Engl J Med* 1983;308:733–740.
44. Benach JL, Bosler EM, Hanrahan JP, et al. Spirochetes isolated from the blood of two patients with Lyme disease. *N Engl J Med* 1983;308:740–742.
45. Burgdorfer W, Lane RS, Barbour AG, Gresbrink RA, Anderson JR. The western black-legged tick, *Ixodes pacificus*: A vector of *Borrelia burgdorferi*. *Am J Trop Med Hyg* 1985;34:925–930.
46. Barbour AG, Burgdorfer W, Hayes SF, Peter O, Aeschlimann A. Isolation of a cultivable spirochete from *Ixodes ricinus* ticks of Switzerland. *Curr Microbiol* 1983;8:123–126.
47. Berger BW, Clemmensen OJ, Ackerman AB. Lyme disease is a spirochetosis. *Am J Dermatopathol* 1983;5:111–124.
48. Asbrink E, Hederstedt B, Hovmark A. The spirochetal etiology of erythema chronicum migrans Afzelius. *Acta Derm Venereol (Stockh)* 1984;64:291–295.
49. Pfister H, Einhaupl K, Preac-Mursic V, Wilske B, Schierz G. The spirochetal etiology of lymphocytic meningoradiculitis of Bannwarth (Bannwarth's syndrome). *J Neurol* 1984;231:141–144.
50. Preac-Mursic V, Wilske B, Schierz G, Pfister HW, Einhaupl K. Repeated isolation of spirochetes from the cerebrospinal fluid of a patient with meningoradiculitis Bannwarth. *Eur J Clin Microbiol* 1984;3:564–565.
51. Frithz A, Lagerholm B. Acrodermatitis chronica atrophicans, erythema chronicum migrans and lymphadenosis benigna cutis—spirochetal diseases? *Acta Derm Venereol (Stockh)* 1983;63:432–436.
52. Hovmark A, Åsbrink E, Olsson I. The spirochetal etiology of lymphadenosis benigna cutis solitaria. *Acta Derm Venereol (Stockh)* 1986;66:479–484.
53. Åsbrink E, Hovmark A, Hederstedt B. The spirochetal etiology of acrodermatitis chronica atrophicans Herxheimer. *Acta Derm Venereol (Stockh)* 1984;64:506–512.
54. Johnson RC, Schmid GP, Hyde FW, Steigerwalt AG, Brenner DJ. *Borrelia burgdorferi* sp. nov.: Etiologic agent of Lyme disease. *Int J Syst Bacteriol* 1984;34:496–497.
55. Reik L, Burgdorfer W, Donaldson JO. Neurologic abnormalities in Lyme disease without erythema chronicum migrans. *Am J Med* 1986;81:73–78.
56. Reik L, Smith L, Khan A, Nelson W. Demyelinating encephalopathy in Lyme disease. *Neurology* 1985;32:1302–1305.
57. Ackermann R, Rehse-Küpper B, Gollmer E. Progressive *Borrelia* encephalomyelitis. *Zentralbl Bakteriol Mikrobiol Hyg [A]* 1986;263:297–300.
58. Halperin JJ, Little BW, Coyle PK, Dattwyler RJ. Lyme disease: Cause of a treatable peripheral neuropathy. *Neurology* 1987;37:1700–1706.
59. Halperin JJ, Pass HL, Anand AK, Luft BJ, Volkman DJ, Dattwyler RJ. Nervous system abnormalities in Lyme disease. *Ann NY Acad Sci* 1988;539:24–34.
60. Steere AC. Lyme disease. *N Engl J Med* 1989;321:586–596.
61. Luft BJ, Gorevic PD, Halperin JJ, Volkman DJ, Dattwyler RJ. A perspective on the treatment of Lyme borreliosis. *Rev Infect Dis* 1989;11(suppl 6):S1518–S1525.
62. Luft BJ, Dattwyler RJ. Treatment of Lyme borreliosis. *Rheum Dis Clin North Am* 1989;15:747–755.

2

Epidemiology and Vectors

Lyme disease has been reported from five continents—Africa, Asia, Australia, Europe, and North America.[1-5] Although other ticks or even flies or other biting insects may transmit the disease in some areas, the usual vectors are small, hard-bodied ticks of the genus *Ixodes*.[6-7] *Ixodes* species have a three-stage (larva, nymph, adult), three-host life cycle, and take a single blood meal during each stage of development, active feeding usually beginning with the onset of warmer weather in early spring.[6] Since the brushy understories of forests and their margins are the preferred habitat of these ticks, the symptoms of Lyme disease begin most often in late spring or summer in individuals exposed to such areas.

Lyme Disease in North America

In North America, Lyme disease occurs in both the United States and Canada. Within the United States, it is now the most commonly reported tick-transmitted infection (4507 cases reported to the Centers for Disease Control in 1988),[1] and it has been acquired in 43 states in all (Figure 2–1).[8] The disease is endemic along the East Coast from Maryland to Massachusetts, in the upper Midwest in Minnesota and Wisconsin, and on the Pacific coast in California and Oregon.[1,2,8] Increasing numbers of cases have also been reported from mid-Atlantic, southeastern, midwestern, and southcentral states. But the illness remains most common in the states from which it was originally reported: In 1987–1988, 92% of the reported cases were from New York, New Jersey, Pennsylvania, Connecticut, Massachusetts, Rhode Island, Wisconsin, and Minnesota.[8] New York reported the most cases (57% of the

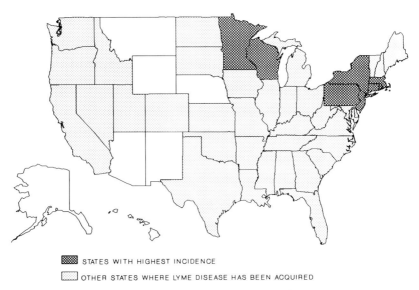

STATES WITH HIGHEST INCIDENCE

OTHER STATES WHERE LYME DISEASE HAS BEEN ACQUIRED

Figure 2–1. Distribution of Lyme disease in the United States, by state of acquisition as of 1988.

national total in 1988), while the incidence was highest in Rhode Island (9.9 cases/100,000).[8]

Lyme disease is less common in Canada.[9,10] Only 30 cases were reported to Canada's Laboratory Centre for Disease Control between 1977 and May 1989, and 5 of those were acquired outside the country.[9] Since Lyme disease is a reportable condition only in Ontario, and since 16 of the 30 reported cases occurred in 1988, it is likely that with increased awareness and more intense surveillance, Lyme disease will prove to be more widespread and common in Canada than it is now known to be. At present, the areas of Canada with the most indigenous cases, Ontario (17 cases) and Manitoba (5 cases), border the American states with the highest reported incidence.[9]

The usual vector in the Northeast and Midwest is the deer tick, *Ixodes dammini* (Color Plates 2–1 and 2–2, page 129). This species ranges along the Atlantic coast from southern Delaware to Massachusetts, and it is common in Wisconsin, Minnesota, and southern Ontario, Canada (Figure 2–2).[6,7,11] The tick also has been collected in upstate New York, New Hampshire, Maine, Ohio, Illinois, and Manitoba, Canada;[7,9,12] and it is likely that the population is continuous from the Atlantic to Manitoba.[7] In some areas, as many as 80% of the ticks are infected with spirochetes,[13] explaining the very high attack rate of Lyme disease in these localities.

I. dammini develops in a 2-year life cycle, and all three of its stages may bite humans.[6,7,14,15] However, immature ticks usually feed on a variety of wild birds and small mammals, especially the white-footed mouse, *Peromyscus leucopus*, while adult ticks feed on larger mammals, particularly the

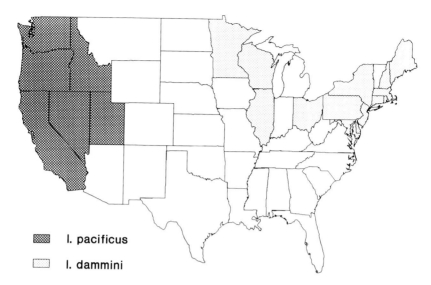

Figure 2–2. Geographic distribution of the major North American vectors of Lyme disease, *Ixodes dammini* and *Ixodes pacificus*, in the United States by state.

white-tailed deer, *Odocoileus virginianus*.[6,7,14–17] Larger domestic animals are parasitized also, and Lyme disease has been reported in dogs, cattle, and horses.[18–20] In all, the ticks have been found to parasitize at least 31 mammalian species and 49 species of birds.[14]

However, it is the presence of both deer and, especially, mice in the environment that is critical for the maintenance of disease transmission. Transovarial transmission of *Borrelia burgdorferi* in *I. dammini* is rare.[21] The infection is maintained in nature instead by horizontal transmission from nymph to larvae through white-footed mice: The nymphs feed on and infect mice from May to July, and the larvae feed on the same mice in August and are infected in turn.[15] Although the mice themselves are readily infected when bitten, they appear to suffer no pathology.[22] Yet they can remain spirochetemic throughout the summer after being infected in the spring and are thus highly infectious to larval ticks for most of their life. The importance of white-footed mice as a reservoir of *B. burgdorferi* is apparent in their high rate of infection: In some areas almost 90% of the mice harbor spirochetes.[17]

The deer, on the other hand, probably serve no reservoir function for natural infection, but as the preferred host for adult ticks they are also critical for the ticks' reproductive success. The elimination of deer in an established focus is followed by a reduced abundance of immature *I. dammini*.[23,24] Consequently, Lyme disease is most frequent in forested and suburban areas where both deer and mice are common.[25]

Larval ticks are infected during the summer by feeding on a spirochetemic host. The ingested organisms then proliferate but remain confined to the midgut. Following feeding, the larvae molt to the nymphal stage (the stage most often involved in transmission to humans) and feed again the following spring. When the nymphs feed, the spirochetes multiply, penetrate the gut wall to enter the hemocele, and disseminate. The salivary glands are invaded, and transmission to the new host then occurs through either infected saliva or the regurgitation of gut contents.[6,26] As the process of dissemination generally takes some time, infection of the new host is likely only if the tick has been attached for more than 24 hours.[27]

In areas where *I. dammini* is common, it clearly is the principal vector of Lyme disease, but other ticks and biting insects may be secondary vectors in parts of its range. In the Northeast, *B. burgdorferi* has also been isolated from the ticks *Dermacentor variabilis*, *Amblyomma americanum*, and *Haemaphysalis leporispalustris* and from horse flies, deer flies, and mosquitoes.[16,28]

On the Pacific coast, the main vector is *Ixodes pacificus*, the western black-legged tick,[6,7,29,30] although the Pacific Coast tick, *Dermacentor occidentalis*, may be a secondary vector in some areas.[30] *I. pacificus* is found in coastal areas from the California-Mexico border to southwestern British Columbia in Canada, and it is also found inland on the western slopes of the Sierra Nevada and Cascade Mountains and in Idaho, Nevada, and Utah (see Figure 2–2).[6,7,11]

I. pacificus develops in a 1-year, three-stage life cycle and, like *I. dammini*, has a wide host range: The tick has been found on approximately 80 species of animals in all.[7] The larvae and nymphs feed on a variety of small mammals, reptiles, and birds while the adults feed on large and medium-size mammals, especially deer, cattle, and wild and domestic canids.[6,7] In California, all stages of *I. pacificus* are active throughout the year, but the adults are most abundant in fall and winter and the nymphs and larvae in spring and early summer. The adults most often bite humans.[7] Because fewer than 3% of these ticks harbor spirochetes in most localities,[29,30] Lyme disease is less common on the West Coast than in areas where *I. dammini* is the vector. The mechanics of disease transmission are probably the same for the two vectors, however, although disseminated infection and transovarial transmission apparently are more frequent in *I. pacificus*.[26]

The vectors in other parts of the United States where Lyme disease has been acquired are less certain. One possible carrier is the common black-legged tick, *Ixodes scapularis*. This widespread tick ranges from Florida, west to Texas, and north to Kansas, Missouri, Iowa, Illinois, Indiana, Ohio, West Virginia, and Maryland (Figure 2–3).[6,7,11] It too has a wide host range: Juveniles feed on a variety of small mammals, birds, and reptiles, particularly lizards, and adults feed on large mammals such as deer, cattle, and swine. All three stages may attack humans, although adult females most often do so.[7] *I. scapularis* can acquire, maintain, and transmit *B. burgdorferi* infection in the laboratory,[31,32] and the organism has been isolated from *I. scapularis* from North Carolina.[33] But it is not clear how often *I. scapularis* actually is a vector of Lyme disease: In Texas, *B. burgdorferi* was isolated from a variety of other

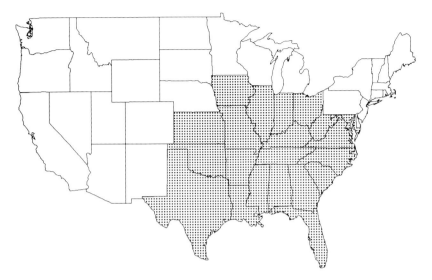

Figure 2–3. Geographic distribution of *Ixodes scapularis* in the United States by state.

ticks collected off infected humans or from sites where human infection was acquired, but not from *I. scapularis* from the same sites.[34]

Lyme Disease in Europe

Lyme disease is both widespread and common in Europe where thousands of cases are estimated to occur each year.[2,35] The disease is most common in Austria, Germany, France, Sweden, and Switzerland. But is also occurs in the three other Scandinavian countries, Belgium, Czechoslovakia, Hungary, Italy, the Netherlands, Romania, Spain, the United Kingdom, the USSR, and Yugoslavia.[2,35]

The main European vector is the sheep tick, *Ixodes ricinus.*[2,6,7,36] *I. ricinus* is found from the British Isles in the west to the Caspian Sea and northern Iran in the east, and from southern Scandinavia in the north to Spain, Portugal, Italy, the Balkans, and North Africa in the south (Figure 2–4).[2,6,7] It occurs in secondary deciduous forests, particularly on their brushy margins, and in clearings with tall grass (pastures).[7,36] *I. ricinus* parasitizes many small mammals, birds, and reptiles as a juvenile, and larger wild and domestic animals as an adult.[6,7] Peak feeding activity for nymphs and adults is in the spring and in the fall. The mechanisms of transmission are probably the same as with *I. dammini*, but *I. ricinus* may, like *I. pacificus*, itself serve as a reservoir for *B. burgdorferi* as transovarial transmission does take place.[37] The infection rate for *I. ricinus* ranges from 5 to 35% in areas where Lyme disease is common,[2] intermediate between those of *I. pacificus* and *I. dammini*.

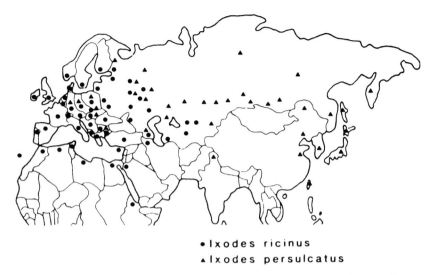

• I x o d e s   r i c i n u s
▲ I x o d e s   p e r s u l c a t u s

Figure 2–4.   Geographic distribution of *Ixodes ricinus* and *Ixodes persulcatus*, the major European and Asian vectors of Lyme disease. (Reproduced with permission from Anderson JF. *Rev Infect Dis* 1989;11(suppl 6):S1451–S1459. Copyright by University of Chicago Press.)

Lyme Disease in Africa, Asia, and Australia

Less is known about the frequency, distribution, and vectors of Lyme disease elsewhere in the world. In Africa, a well-documented case has been reported from Algeria,[5] within the known range of *I. ricinus*, and one from South Africa has been suspected on serologic grounds.[38] In Australia, the disease has been reported from several localities in New South Wales, including the Hunter Valley and the Central and South Coasts.[2,39] Ixodid ticks apparently do occur in Australia,[40] but the vector there has not yet been identified.

Recent reports do suggest that the disease is common in Asia, however. Over 300 cases have been reported in Chinese forest workers from north-central Manchuria near the Sino-Soviet border (Heilongjiang Province),[3] 16 of 90 cases reported from the USSR were from the southern part of the forest zone in Asiatic Russia,[4] and one additional case has been reported from Japan.[41]

The vector in Asia is the taiga tick, *Ixodes persulcatus*.[6,7] This tick is found in a broad band from the Baltic coast of Germany in the east, across eastern Europe and through Asia to Japan (see Figure 2–4). In the east, its range overlaps with that of *I. ricinus*. *I. persulcatus* is found most often in small-leaved deciduous forests and, like its relatives, feeds on a variety of wild and domestic animals. Juvenile ticks parasitize small mammals and birds while adults attack cattle, wild ungulates, lagomorphs, and hedgehogs. All stages feed most actively in late spring and early summer.[6,7]

References

1. Centers for Disease Control. Lyme disease—United States, 1987 and 1988. *MMWR* 1989;38:668–672.
2. Schmid GP. The global distribution of Lyme disease. *Rev Infect Dis* 1985;7:41–50.
3. Chengxu A, Yuxin W, Yongguo Z, et al. Clinical manifestations and epidemiological characteristics of Lyme disease in Hailin County, Heilongjiang Province, China. *Ann NY Acad Sci* 1988;539:302–313.
4. Dekonenko EJ, Steere AC, Berardi VP, Kravchuk LN. Lyme borreliosis in the Soviet Union: A cooperative US-USSR report. *J Infect Dis* 1989;158:748–753.
5. Rousselle C, Floret D, Cochat P, Reignier F, Wright C. Encéphalite aiguë à *Borrelia burgdorferi* (maladie de Lyme) chez un enfant algérien. *Pediatrie* 1989;44:265–269.
6. Burgdorfer W. Vector/host relationships of the Lyme disease spirochete, *Borrelia burgdorferi*. *Rheum Dis Clin North Am* 1989;15:775–787.
7. Anderson JF. Epizootiology of *Borrelia* in *Ixodes* tick vectors and reservoir hosts. *Rev Infect Dis* 1989;11(suppl 6):S1451–S1459.
8. Tsai TF, Bailey RE, Moore PS. National surveillance of Lyme disease, 1987–1988. *Conn Med* 1989;53:324–326.
9. Centers for Disease Control. Lyme disease—Canada. *MMWR* 1989;38:677–678.
10. Lyme disease in Canada. *Can Med Assoc J* 1988;139:233–234. Epidemiologic report.
11. Burgdorfer W, Keirans JE. Ticks and Lyme disease in the United States. *Ann Intern Med* 1983;99:121.
12. Society for Vector Ecology. Regional reports. *Vector Ecol Newslett* 1990;21:4–12.
13. Johnson SE, Klein GC, Schmid GP, Bowen GS, Feeley JC, Schulze T. Lyme disease: A selective medium for isolation of the suspected etiological agent, a spirochete. *J Clin Microbiol* 1984;19:81–82.
14. Anderson JF. Ecology of Lyme disease. *Conn Med* 1989;53:343–346.
15. Spielman A, Levine JF, Wilson ML. Vectorial capacity of North America *Ixodes* ticks. *Yale J Biol Med* 1984;57:507–513.
16. Anderson JF, Magnarelli LA. Avian and mammalian hosts for spirochete-infected ticks and insects in a Lyme disease focus in Connecticut. *Yale J Biol Med* 1984;57:621–641.
17. Anderson JF. Mammalian and avian reservoirs for *B. burgdorferi*. *Ann NY Acad Sci* 1988; 539:180–191.
18. Bosler EM, Cohen DP, Schulze TL, Olsen C, Bernard W, Lissman B. Host responses to *Borrelia burgdorferi* in dogs and horses. *Ann NY Acad Sci* 1988;539:221–234.
19. Burgess EC. *Borrelia burgdorferi* infection in Wisconsin horses and cows. *Ann NY Acad Sci* 1988;539:235–243.
20. Cohen D, Bosler EM, Bernard W, Meirs D, Eisner R, Schulze T. Epidemiologic studies of Lyme disease in horses and their public health significance. *Ann NY Acad Sci* 1988;539: 244–257.
21. Burgdorfer W, Hayes SF, Benach JL. Development of *Borrelia burgdorferi* in ixodid tick vectors. *Ann NY Acad Sci* 1988;539:172–179.
22. Levine JF, Wilson ML, Spielman A. Mice as reservoirs of the Lyme disease spirochete. *Am J Trop Med Hyg* 1985;34:355–360.
23. Wilson ML, Telford SR III, Piesman J, Spielman A. Reduced abundance of immature *Ixodes dammini* (Acari: Ixodidae) following elimination of deer. *J Med Entomol* 1988;25:224–228.
24. Spielman A. Prospects for suppressing transmission of Lyme disease. *Ann NY Acad Sci* 1988;539:212–220.
25. Schulze TL, Parkin WE, Bosler EM. Vector tick populations and Lyme disease: A summary of control strategies. *Ann NY Acad Sci* 1988;539:204–211.
26. Burgdorfer W, Hayes SF, Benach JL. Development of *Borrelia burgdorferi* in ixodid tick vectors. *Ann NY Acad Sci* 1988;539:172–179.
27. Piesman J, Mather TN, Sinsky RJ, Spielman A. Duration of tick attachment and *Borrelia burgdorferi* transmission. *J Clin Microbiol* 1987;25:557–558.
28. Magnarelli LA, Anderson JF, Barbour AG. The etiologic agent of Lyme disease in deer flies, horse flies and mosquitoes. *J Infect Dis* 1986;154:355–358.
29. Burgdorfer W, Lane RS, Barbour AG, Gresbrink RA, Anderson JR. The western black-legged tick, *Ixodes pacificus*: A vector of *Borrelia burgdorferi*. *Am J Trop Med Hyg* 1985;34: 925–930.

30. Lane RS, Lavoie PE. Lyme borreliosis in California: Acarological, clinical, and epidemiological studies. *Ann NY Acad Sci* 1988;539:192–203.
31. Burgdorfer W, Gage KL. Susceptibility of the black-legged tick, *Ixodes scapularis*, to the Lyme disease spirochete, *Borrelia burgdorferi*. *Zentralbl Bakteriol Mikrobiol Hyg [A]* 1986;263:15–20.
32. Piesman J, Sinsky RJ. Ability of *Ixodes scapularis*, *Dermacentor variabilis*, and *Amblyomma americanum* (Acari: Ixodidae) to acquire, maintain, and transmit Lyme disease spirochetes (*Borrelia burgdorferi*). *J Med Entomol* 1988;25:336–339.
33. Magnarelli LA, Anderson JF, Apperson CS, Fish D, Johnson RC, Chappell WA. Spirochetes in ticks and antibodies to *Borrelia burgdorferi* in white-tailed deer from Connecticut, New York State and North Carolina. *J Wildl Dis* 1986;22:178–188.
34. Rawlings JA. Lyme disease in Texas. *Zentralbl Bakteriol Mikrobiol Hyg [A]* 1986;263:483–487.
35. Stanek G, Pletschette M, Flamm H, et al. European Lyme borreliosis. *Ann NY Acad Sci* 1988;539:274–282.
36. Radda A, Burger I, Stanek G, Wewalka G. Austrian hard ticks as vectors of *Borrelia burgdorferi*. *Zentralbl Bakteriol Mikrobiol Hyg [A]* 1986;263:79–82.
37. Stanek G, Burger I, Hirschl A, Wewalka G, Radda A. *Borrelia* transfer by ticks during their life cycle: Studies on laboratory animals. *Zentralbl Bakteriol Mikrobiol Hyg [A]* 1986;263:29–33.
38. Stanek G, Hirschl A, Sternberger H, Wewalka G, Wiedermann G. Does Lyme borreliosis also occur in tropical and subtropical areas? *Zentralbl Bakteriol Mikrobiol Hyg [A]* 1986;236:491–495.
39. Lawrence RH, Bradbury R, Cullen JS. Lyme disease on the NSW central coast. *Med J Aust* 1986;145:364.
40. Steere AC. Lyme disease. *N Engl J Med* 1989;321:586–596.
41. Kawabata M, Baba S, Iguchi K, Yamaguti N, Russell H. Lyme disease in Japan and its possible incriminated tick vector, *Ixodes persulcatus*. *J Infect Dis* 1987;156:854.

3

Borrelia burgdorferi

Borrelia burgdorferi belongs to the eubacterial order Spirochaetales, an order that comprises two families and six genera of helical bacteria with common morphologic features.[1,2] Three of the genera, *Treponema*, *Leptospira*, and *Borrelia*, contain organisms pathogenic for humans and animals. Among these, *Borrelia* species are the longest and most loosely coiled,[3] and they are the only pathogenic spirochetes transmitted to vertebrates by hematophagous arthropods.[1,2]

  B. burgdorferi is the longest (10 to 30 μ) and narrowest (0.2 to 0.3 μ) of the borreliae and it has the fewest flagella (7 to 12 compared to 15 to 30 in other species).[4-7] Like other borreliae, it stains with Giemsa stain[8] and can be demonstrated in tissues by silver impregnation techniques (Figure 3–1),[9,10] and it shares with the other members of its genus the typical spirochetal structure (Figure 3–2).[1,2,4,11] This consists of an outermost, loosely attached, carbohydrate-containing slime layer surrounding a trilaminar outer cell membrane that surrounds in turn the several layers of the protoplasmic cylinder: the outer bacterial cell wall, composed of peptidoglycan; the cytoplasmic membrane, interior to the cell wall; and the enclosed cytoplasmic and nuclear contents. Several periplasmic flagella (axial filaments), responsible for motility, are located between the outer cell membrane and the protoplasmic cylinder. These are attached subterminally to the protoplasmic cylinder at each end; their unattached terminals wrap around the cylinder, extend toward the opposite end of the cell, and overlap at the middle with those from the other end.

  B. burgdorferi also resembles other borreliae in its metabolism and growth requirements.[1,4] The organism seems to prefer an extracellular existence, and it can be grown in culture in complex artificial media (Barbour-Stoenner-

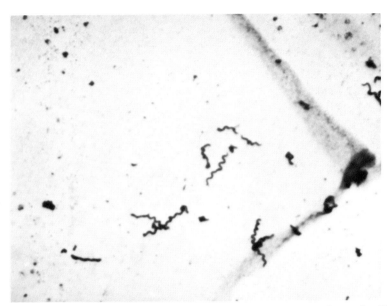

Figure 3–1. *Borrelia burgdorferi* strain B31 stained with the Warthin Starry silver stain. (Photography courtesy of Dr. Alan MacDonald, Department of Pathology, Southampton Hospital, Southampton, NY.)

Kelly, or BSK, medium).[12] Repeated passage in culture (usually 10 to 15) results in loss of infectivity, however.[1,3,13] The growth of laboratory strains in BSK is optimum between 30 and 37°C, yet the organism can remain alive for several months in BSK medium kept at 4°C.[14] At 35°C, the doubling time of laboratory strains is about 12 hours.[15] Some other strains may grow much more slowly: In one recent study, cultures of biopsied specimens from EM lesions became positive by dark-field examination only after prolonged incubation, as long as 10.5 months in some cases.[16]

The organism is catalase negative, microaerophilic, and insensitive to micronidazole. It ferments glucose to lactate via the Embden-Myerhof pathway; incorporates N-acetylglucosamine into peptidoglycan; and requires long-chain fatty acids, which it incorporates unchanged, along with exogenous cholesterol, into cellular lipids.[1,4] Some of this lipid is in the form of a lipopolysaccharide (LPS)[17] which may be the source of endotoxin-like activity.[18] The LPS is located in the outer cell membrane, constitutes between 1.5 and 4% of the dry weight of the organism, and resembles rough-form, gram-negative bacterial LPS.[17] It is mitogenic for human and murine lymphocytes, is pyrogenic for rabbits, produces cross-tolerance to unrelated LPS from *Escherichia coli*, induces the production of interleukin-1 (IL-1), and fails to initiate complement activation.[17]

All isolates of *B. burgdorferi* examined so far have been shown by DNA hybridization to belong to a single species of *Borrelia*,[4,7,19] although some

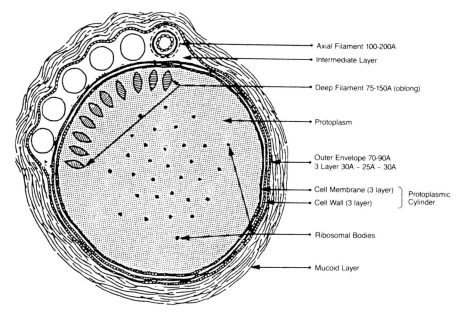

Axial Filament 100-200A
Intermediate Layer
Deep Filament 75-150A (oblong)
Protoplasm
Outer Envelope 70-90A
3 Layer 30A – 25A – 30A
Cell Membrane (3 layer)
Cell Wall (3 layer)
Protoplasmic Cylinder
Ribosomal Bodies
Mucoid Layer

Figure 3–2. Cross-sectional diagram of a spirochete containing six axial filaments (flagella). (Reproduced with permission from Weigand SE, Strobel PL, Glassman LH. *J Invest Dermatol* 1972;58:186–204. Copyright by Williams and Wilkins.)

genetic heterogeneity among isolates has been demonstrated by restriction endonuclease analysis and DNA hybridization of nuclear DNA.[20] In one study,[7] DNA hybridization of ten isolates from the United States and Europe showed a divergence of only 0.0 to 0.1% and a relatedness of 58 to 98%. *B. burgdorferi* DNA contains about 30 mol % of guanine and cytosine, like that of other borreliae,[1,3,4] and it is 30 to 58% homologous with that of North American relapsing fever borreliae, but it is only 16% homologous with treponemal and 1% with leptospiral DNA.[7]

A number of different strains of *B. burgdorferi* have been identified on the basis of variations in their proteins, however.[7,21–29] Polyacrylamide gel electrophoresis and immunoblot analysis of these proteins have shown that all strains tested so far share two components of constant molecular mass, a 60-kd common antigen that is strongly immunogenic and cross-reactive with an equivalent antigen from a wide range of remotely related bacteria,[30] and a 41-kd flagellar antigen that is similar to the flagellar antigens of other spirochetes.[1,3] But the strains vary in several proteins of the outer surface membrane: 31- to 32-kd outer surface protein A (osp A), 33- to 36-kd outer surface protein B (osp B), and 21- to 22-kd protein C (pC).[7,21–29] These three proteins can vary slightly in molecular size and antigenicity and can occur alone or in combination in an individual strain. In the most extensive strain analysis published so far,[26] Wilske and colleagues tested 34 isolates from Europe and North America using polyclonal and monoclonal antibodies against these proteins in immunoblots and were able to define a total of seven different serotypes, five from patients and two from tick isolates.

In general, most North American strains share a similar osp A and differ from each other mainly in their osp B, although a few North American isolates have not reacted with monoclonal antibodies to osp A at all.[7,27] European isolates, on the other hand, are antigenically more diverse, vary more in their osp A than do North American isolates, and differ also in often having a prominent pC, suggesting that *B. burgdorferi* originated in Europe and spread later to North America.[22] Since the 11 European skin isolates tested by Wilske and coworkers were all of the same serotype,[26] it is possible that certain *B. burgdorferi* serotypes cause specific illness patterns, and strain differences may underlie some of the reported clinical differences between North American and European patients with Lyme disease. European CSF isolates are heterogeneous, however.[26]

One way in which variations in outer surface proteins could determine the illness pattern in Lyme disease is through an effect on host cell–parasite interaction and cell adhesion. Borreliae are attracted to, and said to have "tropism" for, certain tissues in their vectors and vertebrate hosts.[1] In ticks, they adhere to midgut epithelial cells[31] and are found in large numbers in neural tissue, salivary glands, and reproductive organs.[1] They seem to be attracted to these tissues by a chemical substance, perhaps an oligosaccharide.[1] In infected vertebrates, *B. burgdorferi*, like other borreliae, has a tendency to settle in the brain,[1] and, *in vitro*, it has been shown to adhere to both neuroglia and their extracellular matrix.[32] The organism also attaches to a variety of other types of mammalian cells in tissue culture (Figure 3–3), including epithelial and endothelial cells and lymphocytes.[31,33,34] If specific outer surface proteins are involved in the spirochete's adhesion to host cells and tissues, then variations in these proteins could result in strain-specific tissue tropisms. In the case of neuroglia, blocking osp A and B with monoclonal antibodies does not alter adherence,[32] so other surface molecules are probably involved; but the adherence of *B. burgdorferi* to cultured endothelial cells is partially blocked by monoclonal antibodies to osp B and to the 41-kd flagellar antigen.[34]

Heterogeneity of surface proteins also occurs in relapsing fever borreliae, and the appearance of new antigenic variants of these proteins in successive generations of spirochetes is thought to be the mechanism through which these organisms escape the host's immune response and produce repeated spirochetemias.[1] Changes in *B. burgdorferi* outer surface proteins have been observed among different generations of the same strain in culture, sometimes occurring at the same time infectivity is lost during serial passage.[15,21,23,26,35] Antigenic variation has also been seen in experimentally infected rabbits that experience recurrent spirochetemias.[36] Indirect evidence suggests that antigenic variation also occurs in human infections. Two European patients with neuroborelliosis have had specific immunoglobulin M (IgM) antibodies against outer surface proteins detectable only by

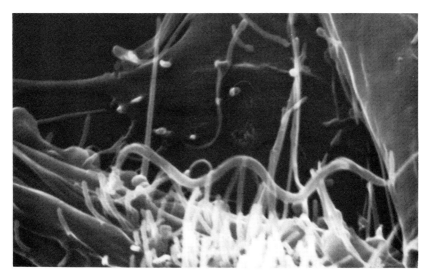

Figure 3–3. Scanning electron micrograph of *Borrelia burgdorferi* adherent to African green monkey kidney cell in culture. (Photograph courtesy of Rocky Mountain Laboratories, National Institute of Allergy and Infectious Diseases, Hamilton, MT.)

reaction with strains antigenically different from their own CSF isolates,[26] presumably because the proteins had changed during the course of infection. In another European case, two different strains were isolated from the CSF of the same patients at 3 and 10 weeks after the onset of neurologic signs.[21]

In addition to nuclear DNA, *B. burgdorferi* contains four to seven different plasmids (pieces of extrachromosomal DNA), both of the usual supercoiled type and of a unique linear variety with covalently closed ends.[1,37–40] The heterogeneity of *B. burgdorferi* outer surface proteins is probably a reflection of the extreme variability of these plasmids among isolates. The genes coding for osp A and osp B are located on a single linear plasmid that operates as a single translational unit.[38] North American strains are congruent for a 49-kilobase (kb) plasmid that contains these genes, while European strains are congruent for a larger 53-kb plasmid coding for the same proteins, but only 2 of 13 strains examined so far have had identical plasmid profiles.[40] Moreover, strains passaged in culture have been shown to lose plasmids at the same time that both outer surface proteins and infectivity are lost,[15] suggesting that all three events may be related.

References

1. Barbour AG, Hayes SF. Biology of *Borrelia* species. *Microbiol Rev* 1986;50:381–400.
2. Schmid GP. Epidemiology and clinical similarities of human spirochetal diseases. *Rev Infect Dis* 1989;11(suppl 6):S1460–S1469.

3. Steere, AC. Lyme disease. *N Engl J Med* 1989;321:586–596.
4. Johnson RC, Hyde FW, Rumpel CM. Taxonomy of the Lyme disease spirochetes. *Yale J Biol Med* 1984;57:529–537.
5. Hovind-Hougen K. Ultrastructure of spirochetes isolated from *Ixodes ricinus* and *Ixodes dammini*. *Yale J Biol Med* 1984;57:543–548.
6. Hovind-Hougen K, Åsbrink E, Stiernstedt G, Steere AC, Hovmark A. Ultrastructural differences among spirochetes isolated from patients with Lyme disease and related disorders, and from *Ixodes ricinus*. *Zentralbl Bakteriol Mikrobiol Hyg [A]* 1986;263:103–111.
7. Anderson JF, Magnarelli LA, LeFebvre RB, et al. Antigenically variable *Borrelia burgdorferi* isolated from cottontail rabbits and *Ixodes dentatus* in rural and urban areas. *J Clin Microbiol* 1989;27:13–20.
8. Burgdorfer W. Discovery of the Lyme disease spirochete and its relation to tick vectors. *Yale J Biol Med* 1984;57:515–520.
9. de Koning J, Bosma RB, Hoogkamp-Korstanje AA. Demonstration of spirochaetes in patients with Lyme disease with a modified silver stain. *J Med Microbiol* 1987;23:261–267.
10. Duray PH, Kusnitz A, Ryan J. Demonstration of the Lyme disease spirochete by a modified Dieterle stain method. *Lab Med* 1985;16:685–687.
11. Wiegand SE, Strobel PL, Glassman LH. Electron microscopic anatomy of pathogenic *Treponema pallidum*. *J Invest Dermatol* 1972;58:186–204.
12. Barbour AG. Isolation and cultivation of Lyme disease spirochetes. *Yale J Biol Med* 1984;57:521–525.
13. Schwan TG, Burgdorfer W, Garon C. Changes in infectivity and plasmid profile of the Lyme disease spirochete, *Borrelia burgdorferi*, as a result of in vitro cultivation. *Infect Immun* 1988;56:1831–1836.
14. Baranton G, Saint-Girons I. *Borrelia burgdorferi* survival in human blood samples. *Ann NY Acad Sci* 1988;539:444–445.
15. Barbour AG, Burgdorfer W, Hayes SF, Péter O, Aeschlimann A. Isolation of a cultivable spirochete from *Ixodes ricinus* ticks of Switzerland. *Curr Microbiol* 1983;8:123–126.
16. MacDonald AB, Berger BW, Schwan TG. Clinical implications of delayed growth of the Lyme borreliosis spirochete, *Borrelia burgdorferi*. *Acta Trop (Basel)* 1990;48:89–94.
17. Habicht GS, Beck G, Benach JL, Coleman JL. *Borrelia burgdorferi* lipopolysaccharide and its role in the pathogenesis of Lyme disease. *Zentralbl Bakteriol Mikrobiol Hyg [A]* 1986;263: 137–141.
18. Fumarola D, Munno I, Marcuccio C, Miragliotta G. Endotoxin-like activity associated with Lyme disease *Borrelia*. *Zentralbl Bakteriol Mikrobiol Hyg [A]* 1986;263:142–145.
19. Schmid GP, Steigerwalt AG, Johnson S, et al. DNA characterization of Lyme disease spirochetes. *Yale J Biol Med* 1984;57:539–542.
20. LeFebvre RB, Perng GC, Johnson RC. Characterization of *Borrelia burgdorferi* isolates by restriction endonuclease analysis and DNA hybridization. *J Clin Microbiol* 1989;27:636–639.
21. Barbour AG, Tessier SL, Hayes SF. Variation in a major surface protein of Lyme disease spirochetes. *Infect Immun* 1984;45:94–100.
22. Barbour AG, Heiland RA, Howe TR. Heterogeneity of major proteins in Lyme disease borreliae: a molecular analysis of North American and European isolates. *J Infect Dis* 1985;152:478–484.
23. Barbour AG, Schrumpf ME. Polymorphisms of major surface proteins of *Borrelia burgdorferi*. *Zentralbl Bakteriol Mikrobiol Hyg [A]* 1986;263:83–91.
24. Wilske B, Preac-Mursic V, Schierz G. Antigenic heterogeneity of European *Borrelia burgdorferi* strains isolated from patients and ticks. *Lancet* 1985;1:1099.
25. Wilske B, Preac-Mursic V, Schierz G, Busch KV. Immunochemical and immunological analysis of European *Borrelia burgdorferi* strains. *Zentralbl Bakteriol Mikrobiol Hyg [A]* 1986;263:92–102.
26. Wilske B, Preac-Mursic V, Schierz G, Kühbeck R, Barbour AG, Kramer M. Antigenic variability of *Borrelia burgdorferi*. *Ann NY Acad Sci* 1988;539:126–143.
27. Bissett ML, Hill W. Characterization of *Borrelia burgdorferi* strains isolated from *Ixodes pacificus* ticks in California. *J Clin Microbiol* 1987;25:2296–2301.
28. Anderson JF, Magnarelli LA, McAninch JB. New *Borrelia burgdorferi* antigenic variant isolated from *Ixodes dammini* from upstate New York. *J Clin Microbiol* 1988;26:2209–2212.
29. Lane RS, Pascocello JA. Antigenic characteristics of *Borrelia burgdorferi* isolates from ixodid ticks in California. *J Clin Microbiol* 1989;27:2344–2349.

30. Hansen K, Bangsborg JM, Fjordvang H, Pedersen NS, Hindersson P. Immunochemical characterization of and isolation of the gene for a *Borrelia burgdorferi* immunodominant 60-kilodalton antigen common to a wide range of bacteria. *Infect Immun* 1988;56:2047–2053.
31. Benach JL, Coleman JL, Garcia-Monco JC, Deponte PC. Biological activity of *Borrelia burgdorferi* antigens. *Ann NY Acad Sci* 1988;539:115–125.
32. Garcia-Monco JC, Fernandez-Villar B, Benach JL. Adherence of the Lyme disease spirochete to glial cells and cells of glial origin. *J Infect Dis* 1989;160:497–506.
33. Hechemy KE, Samsonoff WA, McKee M, Guttman JM. *Borrelia burgdorferi* attachment to mammalian cells. *J Infect Dis* 1989;159:805–806.
34. Thomas DD, Comstock LE. Interaction of Lyme disease spirochetes with cultured eucaryotic cells. *Infect Immun* 1989;57:1324–1326.
35. Schwan TG, Burgdorfer W. Antigenic changes of *Borrelia burgdorferi* as a result of in vitro cultivation. *J Infect Dis* 1987;156:852–853.
36. Burgdorfer W, Gage KL. Susceptibility of the black-legged tick, *Ixodes scapularis*, to the Lyme disease spirochete, *Borrelia burgdorferi*. *Zentralbl Bakteriol Mikrobiol Hyg [A]* 1986;263:15–20.
37. Barbour AG. The molecular biology of *Borrelia*. *Rev Infect Dis* 1989;11(suppl 6):S1470–S1474.
38. Howe TR, LaQuier FW, Barbour AG. Organization of genes encoding two outer membrane proteins of the Lyme disease agent *Borrelia burgdorferi* within a single transcriptional unit. *Infect Immun* 1986;54:207–212.
39. Barbour AG, Garon CF. The genes encoding major surface proteins of *Borrelia burgdorferi* are located on a plasmid. *Ann NY Acad Sci* 1988;539:144–153.
40. Barbour AG. Plasmid analysis of *Borrelia burgdorferi*, the Lyme disease agent. *J Clin Microbiol* 1988;26:475–478.

4

Pathogenesis and Pathophysiology

Lyme Disease in Animals

Borrelia burgdorferi infection in animals replicates many of the clinical abnormalities of human Lyme disease, but no single animal model replicates them all. Both naturally infected white-footed mice[1] and experimentally infected rabbits[2,3] develop skin lesions and spirochetemia. Experimentally infected laboratory rats[4,5] and irradiated hamsters[6,7] and naturally infected dogs,[8-10] horses,[11-13] and cows[11,14,15] develop arthritis. Infected cows have also had mastitis, spontaneous abortion, myocarditis, interstitial nephritis, glomerulonephritis, and pneumonitis,[11,14,15] while infection in horses has caused swelling of the legs, weight loss, dermatitis, conjunctivitis, panuveitis, nasal discharge, and cough.[11-13]

The organism has also been isolated from the brain of a horse with encephalitis,[16] and both facial palsy and meningitis in dogs have been attributed to *B. burgdorferi* infection.[17] But nervous system infection in other nonhuman hosts has caused only minor histopathologic changes in the brain (microgliosis in hamsters,[18] perivascular mononuclear cell infiltrates in mice[19]), without clinical neurologic abnormalities. In laboratory animals, nervous system infection without symptoms is more usual.

Many laboratory animals can be infected with *B. burgdorferi*, but most show no signs of disease. These include Syrian hamsters,[18,20,21] inbred mice,[19,22] hispid cotton rats,[23] and splenectomized gerbils.[22,24] Among these, the Syrian hamster is the best studied.[18,20,21] In hamsters infected by intradermal inoculation, the organism proliferates locally, quickly enters the blood vessels and lymphatics, and, probably aided by its ability to adhere to and penetrate through and between endothelial cells,[25-27] disseminates to multi-

22

ple organs. Spirochetes can be isolated from the blood of cutaneously infected hamsters as early as the first day of infection. By the fifth day, they are still present in the skin at the original site of inoculation, and they can be either isolated from or visualized histologically in the gonads, lungs, kidneys, and heart. By the seventh day, the organisms are present in the brain and eyes.[18,20] In intravenously infected Lewis rats, *B. burgdorferi* penetrates the blood-brain barrier even earlier, between 12 and 48 hours after inoculation.[28]

Early spirochetemia is also a feature of *B. burgdorferi* infection in other laboratory animals, and, in several of them, there can be repeated waves of spirochetemia as in the relapsing fevers. Such relapses have been observed in experimentally infected rabbits,[29] splenectomized gerbils,[22] hispid cotton rats,[23] and mice.[22]

Once the spirochetes do reach the tissues, they remain mostly extracellular there and can persist for a long time: Hamsters remain infected for as long as 14 months.[18] How long the organisms persist in the central nervous system (CNS) is not known, but Muhlemann and Wright stated that the spirochete can remain dormant in the brain for years in experimental murine borrelial infections.[30] Similarly, Burgdorfer and Gage isolated the related relapsing fever borrelia *Borrelia duttonii* from the brain tissues of Swiss mice 475 days after infection.[23]

The organisms also retain the capacity for bloodstream invasion for a long time. In the hamster, spirochetes have been visualized in heart blood more than 6 months after inoculation,[21] wild white-footed mice can remain spirochetemic for 13 months after they are brought into the laboratory,[31] and experimentally infected dogs have developed spirochetemia after a single dose of dexamethasone given on the 68th day of infection.[32]

It is not clear how *B. burgdorferi* is able to evade the host's immune response and establish persistent infection. Initially, components of the vector tick's saliva may help the organism escape the host's defenses. The saliva of *Ixodes dammini* contains antihemostatic, antiinflammatory, and immunosuppressive elements that facilitate blood-feeding success.[33] These elements include an antiplatelet aggregation factor; an anticoagulant acting on the intrinsic pathway of the coagulation cascade; an apyrase that hydrolyzes ATP and ADP; prostaglandin E_2 (PE_2), which suppresses macrophage activation and neutrophil activity; a kininase that inactivates bradykinin; and an inhibitor of T-cell activation and, therefore, subsequent antibody production. The early action of these factors may allow the spirochetes to proliferate locally, enter the blood vessels, and disseminate without eliciting a local inflammatory or immune response.

Once the organisms disseminate, other mechanisms must operate to protect them from immune attack and elimination, however. As the spirochetes largely remain extracellular, they should be vulnerable to attack. Possible escape mechanisms include sequestration in immunologically privileged sites, antigenic mimicry or variation, and suppression of the host's immune defenses by the spirochete. There is evidence from animal experiments that several of these mechanisms may be operating.

Experimentally infected Syrian hamsters develop specific antibodies against *B. burgdorferi*, but the organism persists in tissues despite the presence of these antibodies. Immunization of Syrian hamsters with inactivated *B. burgdorferi* does protect them against subsequent infection,[34] and passive immunization of hamsters with either rabbit or hamster anti–*B. burgdorferi* antibodies also prevents the animals from being infected with the same strain of spirochete against which the antibodies were raised, but only if the antibodies are administered prior to challenge.[18] Hamsters passively immunized 17 hours after the challenge are not protected,[18] suggesting that the spirochete can be sequestered rapidly in host tissues where it is either resistant to or inaccessible to the protective effect of the antibody.

Passive immunization experiments also suggest that serum immunity to *B. burgdorferi* infection in hamsters is strain specific. Immunization of hamsters against a *B. burgdorferi* isolate from one geographic area does not protect against challenge with an isolate from another geographic area.[18] Among strains of borreliae from different areas, the antigens that elicit formation of protective antibody must be heterogeneous, therefore, suggesting that antigenic shifts in outer surface proteins, if they do occur *in vivo*, could protect the spirochetes from immune elimination.

Even if the immune response is not capable of eliminating the organism, it is nonetheless important in determining the extent and severity of illness and in containing the organism. Immune-suppressed animals develop more severe illness: Only irradiated hamsters develop arthritis after experimental infection,[6,7] neonatal laboratory rats develop arthritis more easily than weanling rats,[4,5] and gerbils must be splenectomized before they can develop measurable spirochetemia while bank voles infected in the wild develop spontaneous spirochetemia after splenectomy in the laboratory.[24]

T-cell responses are also likely to be important in experimental infections, but not much is known about them. An antigen-specific T-cell response does develop in inbred mice experimentally infected with *B. burgdorferi*, is present as early as 10 days after inoculation, and increases over subsequent weeks.[19] The response varies among inbred strains, but the variation is not related to histocompatibility loci (H-2 haplotype), and is probably controlled by other non-H-2 genes. Whether variations in the T-cell response are related to differences in disease susceptibility in animals infected with *B. burgdorferi* is not known at present, however.

Lyme Disease in Humans

Proliferation, Dissemination, and Persistence of B. burgdorferi

In the human host, *B. burgdorferi* also first proliferates locally in the skin at the site of the tick bite where its presence and the host's reaction to it cause the skin lesion, erythema migrans [EM].[35,36] EM develops days to weeks after the infecting tick bite, and the spirochete can be both demonstrated histologically in and cultured from the skin lesion at this early stage.[37,38]

Within days or weeks, the organism spreads hematogenously throughout the body: *B. burgdorferi* has been isolated from the bloodstream as early as 4 days after a tick bite and as soon as 2 days after the appearance of EM.[39,40] It is not known, however, whether repeated waves of spirochetemia can occur in infected humans as they do in laboratory animals. Nor is it known whether the organism similarly retains the capacity for bloodstream invasion in the human host over time.

During dissemination, a prominent immune response develops and is characterized by proliferation of lymphocytes and plasma cells, production of increased levels of IgM, the appearance of circulating immune complexes, and hyperplasia of the reticuloendothelial system.[35] The spirochetes appear to have a predilection for the reticuloendothelial system at this stage, and they can be demonstrated histologically in hyperplastic lymph nodes, spleen, liver, bone marrow, and testis.[36]

If spirochetemia occurs during pregnancy, transplacental transmission can result. Both fetal demise and congenital infection have been reported following maternal Lyme disease during pregnancy, and *B. burgdorferi* has been recovered from and demonstrated in a number of fetal tissues including the liver, heart, kidney, adrenal, meninges, subarachnoid space, and brain.[41–44] However, the tissues generally have not been inflamed, and no consistent pattern of congenital malformation has been linked to intrauterine infection.[45]

One or two months after dissemination, the spirochete seems to localize, becoming sequestered in certain tissues, particularly the nervous system and heart. *B. burgdorferi* has been demonstrated in the brain parenchyma[46,47] and cultured from the CSF of a number of patients with early neurologic involvement[39,48–54]: It has been recovered from CSF as early as 18 days after a tick bite[54] and as long as 9 months after a preceding EM.[49] Moreover, the organism can be demonstrated in the heart, skeletal muscle, and eye, and it is still present in the skin at this stage.[35,36]

Once the organism is sequestered in the tissues, it can persist there, just as it does in infection of laboratory animals. Lyme arthritis develops weeks to years after the onset of illness (mean, 6 months) and can continue for years once it has begun.[55] Even at this late stage, live spirochetes are still present: They have been cultured from joint fluid[56,57] and can be demonstrated histologically in synovium.[58] In addition, other progressive skin and nervous system abnormalities can begin years after the initial infection because of the survival of live organisms. Spirochetes can be demonstrated in and cultured from these late skin lesions as long as 10 years after the onset,[59] and they have been demonstrated by silver staining of CSF sediment as long as 15 months after the beginning of neurologic symptoms.[60] Although *B. burgdorferi* has not been cultured yet from the nervous system in the late stage of disease, the response of late neurologic disease to antibiotics suggests that the organism remains alive there as well.

The Human Immune Response to B. burgdorferi

Persisting *B. burgdorferi* infection in humans occurs in spite of a vigorous cellular and humoral immune response, very much as it does in experimental Lyme disease.

The T-cell response develops first.[61,62] Lymphocytes from patients with Lyme disease proliferate in response to *B. burgdorferi* beginning early in the course of the illness, before there is measurable antibody production; once established, this response is long lasting, not related to disease activity, and unaffected by antibiotic therapy.[63] The reactive mononuclear cells are concentrated at the sites of disease activity—in the synovial fluid of Lyme arthritis patients[64] and in the CSF of patients with early neurologic involvement[65]—suggesting an active response by antigen-specific T cells to *B. burgdorferi* localized in these tissues.[66]

Both the total number of lymphocytes and the number of T cells in patients with Lyme disease is probably normal,[62] although lymphopenia was found to occur early in the illness in one report.[67] But there is evidence that the presence of *B. burgdorferi* alters the host's T-cell response qualitatively as the number of cells in specific T-cell subsets is not normal. The natural killer (NK) cytotoxic ability of peripheral blood lymphocytes is normal in patients with early treated or seronegative disease, but it is below normal in patients with active disease.[62,68] This inhibition of NK function is probably the result of interaction between proliferating organisms and the host immune system since it occurs *in vitro* only in the presence of actively proliferating *B. burgdorferi*, but the mechanism is not clear.[68] Suppressor-cell changes occur also. Suppressor-cell activity is increased early in the illness, then becomes depressed later on, explaining both an initial delay in the appearance of specific antibody and a subsequent vigorous humoral response.[62,69,70]

The human humoral response to *B. burgdorferi* develops more slowly than the T-cell response. Specific antibody is usually not yet detectable when EM appears, the IgM response typically becoming maximum 3 to 6 weeks later and then declining, although titers may remain elevated during severe disease.[71–74] The specific IgM response is often directed at the 41-kd flagellar antigen[72,75] and is frequently accompanied by evidence of polyclonal activation of B cells: elevated total levels of IgM; circulating immune complexes and cryoglobulins containing IgM, immunoglobulin G (IgG), and components of complement; rheumatoid factor; antinuclear antibodies; and anticardiolipin antibodies.[55,66,76]

IgG antibody appears next: Measurable amounts are nearly always present during early neurologic or joint involvement.[39,72] Once specific IgG is present, the antibody can persist in high titer for years, even during remission.[39,72,73] Like the IgM response, the IgG response is directed initially against the 41-kd antigen, but the IgG response expands with time to recognize an increasing number of spirochetal polypeptides.[73,75] This expanding response is not seen in patients with early disease who are treated successfully with antibiotics, and it ceases in patients with late disease once treatment is given.

Immune antibodies facilitate the phagocytosis and killing of *B. burgdorferi* by polymorphonuclear leukocytes (PMNs) and monocytes,[77] and they are necessary for serum-mediated killing of the organism through the classic complement pathway.[78] But the development of humoral immunity neither protects humans from reinfection[79,80] nor does it eradicate *B. burgdorferi* from established infections. The demonstration of spirochetes in and their recovery from patients with high titers of specific antibody and the expansion of the antibody response that ceases with antibiotic treatment of late disease both indicate the presence of live organisms despite high levels of specific antibody.[81]

Disease Mechanisms

Yet *B. burgdorferi* is difficult to isolate from human material, and, when present in tissue, the organisms are sparse and hard to find, suggesting that their harmful effects may be magnified through inflammatory mediators, immunologic mechanisms, or other indirect actions.

B. burgdorferi itself, its outer surface protein A (osp A), and flagellin are all chemotactic for PMNs,[82] while *B. burgdorferi* lipopolysaccharide (LPS) has endotoxin-like activity[83] and can stimulate the release of IL-1 from macrophages.[84,85] IL-1 may mediate many of the general features of Lyme disease: It causes fever, fatigue, anorexia, leukocytosis, and the synthesis of acute-phase reactants. It is also chemotactic for PMNs, stimulates antibody production, and induces lymphocytes to secrete interleukin-2 (IL-2), causing in turn the release of lymphokines and local increases in the number of lymphocytes. IL-1 is found in the joint fluid in Lyme arthritis[86]; within joints, it causes the release of collagenase, proteases, PE_2, and plasminogen activator from chondrocytes and synovial cells.[85,87] Moreover, the intradermal injection of IL-2 in the rabbit has caused EM-like lesions.[84]

Immunopathic tissue damage in response to the presence of the spirochetes may be an additional factor in pathogenesis. Possible mechanisms include the cross-reaction of anti–*B. burgdorferi* antibodies with host antigens, the induction of cellular autoimmunity, the deposition of circulating immune complexes in tissues, and the uncontrolled local production of specific antibody because of the loss of suppressor activity leading to local formation of immune complexes and chronic inflammation.

CENTRAL NERVOUS SYSTEM DISEASE

Both the direct effects of the organism and the host's reaction to it are probably important in causing CNS disease.

Meningitis almost certainly is caused directly by the invasion of the CSF by *B. burgdorferi*, as the spirochete has been cultured from the CSF[39,48–54] and antibiotics shorten the course.[88] Since *B. burgdorferi* also has been demonstrated histologically in and isolated from brain tissue,[46,47] and since late parenchymal CNS disease also responds to antibiotic therapy,[89] at least some CNS parenchymal abnormalities probably result from direct invasion as well.

Yet several lines of clinical evidence suggest that some other CNS abnormalities are due to vasculopathy. These include the diffuse and multifocal pattern of neurologic abnormalities in some patients, the occurrence of apparent transient ischemic attacks and stroke-like episodes in some patients with encephalopathy, the high frequency of hemiparesis in some series, computerized tomographic (CT) abnormalities suggesting cerebral infarction, and cerebral angiographic changes indicative of vasculitis.[90] CNS vasculitis has not been demonstrated histologically, however, and the evidence for it is only indirect, but vasculitis has been seen in other tissues in Lyme disease.[35]

Although the presence of CNS vasculitis in Lyme disease can only be inferred, several mechanisms could operate to produce it. *B. burgdorferi* adheres to and penetrates endothelial cell monolayers[25–27] and adheres to glial cells and their extracellular matrix.[91] The inflammatory response to spirochetes in and around blood vessels in the brain, or the *in situ* formation of immune complexes composed of immunoglobulin and their shed or degraded surface antigens, or both, could be one cause of this putative vasculitis, as could the deposition of circulating immune complexes in cerebral vessel walls. However, *B. burgdorferi* has not been demonstrated in or around vessel walls in the CNS, and immune complexes have not been localized to sites of vascular injury in the CNS or elsewhere. Immune complexes are present in the blood and CSF of many patients with Lyme disease and neurologic abnormalities, however.[92–95]

Other immunopathic mechanisms also may operate to cause CNS disease. CT and magnetic resonance images (MRIs) from some patients with Lyme disease and cerebral symptoms have shown changes consistent with demyelination.[96–98] Moreover, antibodies to both myelin and myelin basic protein have been found in serum and CSF of patients with neurologic abnormalities of Lyme disease,[99,100] and the CSF of some patients with radiculomyelitis contains T-cell lines reactive to myelin basic protein, peripheral myelin, and galactocerebrosides in addition to *B. burgdorferi*–specific T-cell lines.[101]

Cross-reacting antibodies may also contribute to nervous system injury in Lyme disease. The 41-kd flagellar protein shares antigenic determinants with myelinated fibers of human peripheral nerve and with nerve cells and axons of the CNS,[102] and serum from patients with neurologic manifestations of Lyme disease, but not from those without, contains IgM antibodies that bind to normal human axons.[103]

PERIPHERAL NERVOUS SYSTEM DISEASE

Both the direct effect of the organism and the host's reaction to it may contribute to peripheral nervous system (PNS) disease as well. Spinal radiculitis and cranial neuritis could result directly from extension of inflammation from the meninges and subarachnoid space to the nerve roots.[104] Yet some patients with radiculoneuritis do not have pleocytosis, and the clinical patterns typical of early neurologic involvement—mononeuritis simplex and multiplex and asymmetric radiculoplexitis—again suggest a vasculopathy.[90,93] Examination of biopsied nerve specimens has shown vasculopathy in a number of cases,[105–107] and electrophysiologic testing often shows multifocal axonal injury consistent with a vascular cause.[104–106,108]

In other cases, however, the electrophysiologic findings indicate demyelination.[104,109,110] Furthermore, severe weakness in Lyme disease can resolve in weeks,[93,104,111,112] suggesting remyelination after demyelination rather than the slower regeneration that occurs after wallerian degeneration.

Both demyelination and axonal injury occur in the PNS in Lyme disease, therefore. It is possible that both result from the same vasculopathy. The presence of antibodies to myelin and myelin basic protein in serum and CSF of patients with neurologic abnormalities[99,100] and the detection of T-cell lines in their CSF reactive to peripheral myelin[101] suggest that demyelination could result from indirect immunopathologic mechanisms, however.

Immunogenetic Linkage

Presumably these immunologic mechanisms are under genetic control, but the human leukocyte antigen (HLA) linkages to late manifestations of Lyme disease are not clear. Initial reports described an increased incidence of HLA-DRw2 and an increase of DR7 in patients with Lyme arthritis,[113] but further studies have not substantiated this relationship. There does appear to be a relationship between an increase in DR4 and chronic arthritis, however.[114]

Whether there is a histocompatibility linkage to neurologic manifestations in Lyme disease is not certain. In an early study, Kristoferitsch and Mayr[115] found no association between DR2 and meningopolyneuritis in European patients. Subsequently, Wokke et al.[116] also found no correlation between HLA-DR2 and meningopolyneuritis, but they did find that the frequency of DR2 was significantly higher in patients with elevated levels of IgG antibodies against *B. burgdorferi* when tested by indirect immunofluorescence. Majsky et al.,[117] on the other hand, found an association between HLA-DR2 and facial palsy combined with other cranial nerve impairment and between DR4 and radiculitis and myeloradiculitis. To my knowledge, the HLA linkages to other forms of neurologic involvement in Lyme disease have not been studied.

References

1. Magnarelli LA, Anderson JF, Chappell WA. Geographic distribution of humans, raccoons, and white-footed mice with antibodies to Lyme disease spirochetes in Connecticut. *Yale J Biol Med* 1984;57:619–626.
2. Burgdorfer W. The New Zealand White rabbit: An experimental host for infecting ticks with Lyme disease spirochetes. *Yale J Biol Med* 1984;57:609–612.
3. Kornblatt AN, Steere AC, Brownstein DG. Experimental Lyme disease in rabbits: Spirochetes found in erythema migrans and blood. *Infect Immun* 1984;46:220–223.
4. Barthold SW, Moody KD, Terwilliger GA, Jacoby RO, Steere AC. An animal model for Lyme arthritis. *Ann NY Acad Sci* 1988;539:264–273.
5. Barthold SW, Moody KD, Terwilliger GA, Duray PH, Jacoby RO, Steere AC. Experimental Lyme arthritis in rats infected with *Borrelia burgdorferi*. *J Infect Dis* 1988;157:842–846.
6. Schmitz JL, Schell RF, Hejka A, England DM, Konick L. Induction of Lyme arthritis in LSH hamsters. *Infect Immun* 1988;56:2336–2342.
7. Hejka A, Schmitz JL, England DM, Callister SM, Schell RF. Histopathology of Lyme arthritis in LSH hamsters. *Am J Pathol* 1989;134:1113–1123.
8. Lissman BA, Bosler EM, Camay H, Ormiston BG, Benach JL. Spirochete-associated arthritis (Lyme disease) in a dog. *J Am Vet Med Assoc* 1984;185:219–220.
9. Kornblatt AN, Urband PH, Steere AC. Arthritis caused by *Borrelia burgdorferi* in dogs. *J Am Vet Med Assoc* 1985;186:960–964.
10. Magnarelli LA, Anderson JF, Kaufmann AF, Lieberman LL, Whitney GD. Borreliosis in dogs from southern Connecticut. *J Am Vet Med Assoc* 1985;186:955–959.
11. Burgess EC. *Borrelia burgdorferi* infection in Wisconsin horses and cows. *Ann NY Acad Sci* 1988;539:235–243.
12. Bosler EM, Cohen DP, Schulze TL, Olsen C, Bernard W, Lissman B. Host responses to *Borrelia burgdorferi* in dogs and horses. *Ann NY Acad Sci* 1988;539:221–234.
13. Cohen D, Bosler EM, Bernard W, Meirs D, Eisner R, Schulze TL. Epidemiologic studies of Lyme disease in horses and their public health significance. *Ann NY Acad Sci* 1988;539:244–257.
14. Burgess EC, Gendron-Fitzpatrick A, Wright WO. Arthritis and systemic disease caused by *Borrelia burgdorferi* infection in a cow. *J Am Vet Med Assoc* 1987;191:1468–1470.
15. Post JE, Shaw EE, Wright SD. Suspected borreliosis in cattle. *Ann NY Acad Sci* 1988;539:488.
16. Burgess EC, Mattison M. Encephalitis associated with *Borrelia burgdorferi* infection in a horse. *J Am Vet Med Assoc* 1987;191:1457–1458.
17. Mörner AP, Olson P, Carlsson M, Olersbacken M. Clinical and serological studies of borreliosis in Swedish dogs. Presented at the Fourth International Conference on Lyme Borreliosis; June 18–21, 1990; Stockholm, Sweden.
18. Johnson RC, Kodner C, Russell M, Duray P. Experimental infection of the hamster with *Borrelia burgdorferi*. *Ann NY Acad Sci* 1988;539:258–263.
19. Schaible UE, Kramer MD, Justus CWE, Museteanu C, Simon MM. Demonstration of antigen-specific T cells and histopathological alterations in mice experimentally inoculated with *Borrelia burgdorferi*. *Infect Immun* 1989;57:41–47.
20. Johnson RC, Marek N, Kodner C. Infection of Syrian hamsters with Lyme disease spirochetes. *J Clin Microbiol* 1984;20:1099–1101.
21. Duray PH, Johnson RC. The histopathology of experimentally infected hamsters with the Lyme disease spirochete, *Borrelia burgdorferi* (42251). *Proc Soc Exp Biol Med* 1986;181:263–269.
22. Stanek G, Burger I, Hirschl A, Wewalka G, Radda A. *Borrelia* transfer by ticks during their life cycle: studies on laboratory animals. *Zentralbl Bakteriol Mikrobiol Hyg [A]* 1986;263:29–33.
23. Burgdorfer W, Gage KL. Susceptibility of the hispid cotton rat (*Sigmodon hispidus*) to the Lyme disease spirochete (*Borrelia burgdorferi*). *Am J Trop Med Hyg* 1987;37:624–628.
24. Krampitz HE. In vivo isolation and maintenance of wild strains of European hard tick spirochetes in mammalian and arthropod hosts. *Zentralbl Bakteriol Mikrobiol Hyg [A]* 1986;263:21–28.
25. Thomas DD, Comstock LE. Interaction of Lyme disease spirochetes with cultured eucaryotic cells. *Infect Immun* 1989;57:1324–1326.
26. Comstock LE, Thomas DD. Penetration of endothelial cell monolayers by *Borrelia burgdorferi*. *Infect Immun* 1989;57:1626–1628.
27. Szczepanski A, Furie MB, Benach JL, Lane BP, Fleit HB. Interaction between *Borrelia burgdorferi* and endothelium in vitro. *J Clin Invest* 1990;85:1637–1647.

28. Garcia-Monco JC, Szczepanski A, Villar BF, Benach JL. Experimental approaches to the neuropathogenesis of Lyme disease. Presented at the Fourth International Conference on Lyme borreliosis; June 18–21, 1990; Stockholm, Sweden.

29. Burgdorfer W, Gage KL. Susceptibility of the black-legged tick, *Ixodes scapularis*, to the Lyme disease spirochete, *Borrelia burgdorferi*. *Zentralbl Bakteriol Mikrobiol Hyg [A]* 1986;263:15–20.

30. Muhlemann MF, Wright DJM. Emerging pattern of Lyme disease in the United Kingdom and Irish Republic. *Lancet* 1987;1:260–262.

31. Bosler CM, Schulze TL. The prevalence and significance of *Borrelia burgdorferi* in the urine of feral reservoir hosts. *Zentralbl Bakteriol Mikrobiol Hyg [A]* 1986;263:40–44.

32. Burgess EC. Experimental inoculation of dogs with *Borrelia burgdorferi*. *Zentralbl Bakteriol Mikrobiol Hyg [A]* 1986;263:49–54.

33. Ribeiro JMC, Makoul GT, Levine J, Robinson DR, Spielman A. Antihemostatic, antiinflammatory, and immunosuppressive properties of the saliva of a tick, *Ixodes dammini*. *J Exp Med* 1985;161:332–344.

34. Johnson RC, Kodner CL, Russell ME. Vaccination of hamsters against experimental infection with *Borrelia burgdorferi*. *Zentralbl Bakteriol Mikrobiol Hyg [A]* 1986;263:45–48.

35. Duray PH, Steere AC. Clinical pathologic correlations of Lyme disease by stage. *Ann NY Acad Sci* 1988;539:65–79.

36. Duray PH. Clinical pathologic correlations of Lyme disease. *Rev Infect Dis* 1989;11(suppl 6):S1487–S1493.

37. Berger BW, Clemmensen OJ, Ackerman AB. Lyme disease is a spirochetosis. *Am J Dermatopathol* 1983;5:111–124.

38. Berger BW, Kaplan MH, Rothenberg IR, Barbour AG. Isolation and characterization of the Lyme disease spirochete from the skin of patients with erythema chronicum migrans. *J Am Acad Dermatol* 1985;13:444–449.

39. Steere AC, Grodzicki RI, Kornblatt AN, et al. The spirochetal etiology of Lyme disease. *N Engl J Med* 1983;308:733–740.

40. Benach JL, Bosler EM, Hanrahan JP, et al. Spirochetes isolated from the blood of two patients with Lyme disease. *N Engl J Med* 1983;308:740–742.

41. MacDonald AB. Human fetal borreliosis, toxemia of pregnancy, and fetal death. *Zentralbl Bakteriol Mikrobiol Hyg [A]* 1986;263:189–200.

42. MacDonald AB. Gestational Lyme borreliosis: Implications for the fetus. *Rheum Dis Clin North Am* 1989;15:657–677.

43. Schlesinger PA, Duray PH, Burke BA, Steere AC, Stillman MT. Maternal-fetal transmission of the Lyme disease spirochete, *Borrelia burgdorferi*. *Ann Intern Med* 1985;103:67–68.

44. Weber K, Bratzke H-J, Neubert U, Wilske B, Duray PH. *Borrelia burgdorferi* in a newborn despite oral penicillin for Lyme borreliosis during pregnancy. *Pediatr Infect Dis* 1988;7:286–289.

45. Markowitz LE, Steere AC, Benach JL, Slade JD, Broome CV. Lyme disease during pregnancy. *JAMA* 1986;255:3394–3396.

46. Pachner AR, Duray P, Steere AC. Central nervous system manifestations of Lyme disease. *Arch Neurol* 1989;46:790–795.

47. MacDonald AB, Miranda JM. Concurrent neocortical borreliosis and Alzheimer's disease. *Hum Pathol* 1987;18:759–761.

48. Preac-Mursic V, Wilske B, Schierz G, Pfister H-W, Einhäupl K. Repeated isolation of spirochetes from the cerebrospinal fluid of a patient with meningoradiculitis Bannwarth. *Eur J Clin Microbiol* 1984;3:564–565.

49. Preac-Mursic V, Weber K, Pfister H-W, et al. Survival of *Borrelia burgdorferi* in antibiotically treated patients with Lyme borreliosis. *Infection* 1989;17:355–359.

50. Vieyres C, Allal J, Coisne D, Thomas Ph, Neau JP, Breux JP. Aspects européens de la maladie de Lyme: huit cas. *Presse Med* 1987;16:59–62.

51. Huppertz H-I, Sticht-Groh V. Meningitis due to *Borrelia burgdorferi* in the initial stage of Lyme disease. *Eur J Pediatr* 1989;148:428–430.

52. Rawlings J, Fournier PV, Teltow GJ. Isolation of *Borrelia* spirochetes from patients in Texas. *J Clin Microbiol* 1987;25:1148–1150.

53. Pfister H-W, Preac-Mursic V, Wilske B, Einhäupl K-M, Weinberger K. Latent Lyme neuroborreliosis: Presence of *Borrelia burgdorferi* in the cerebrospinal fluid without concurrent inflammatory signs. *Neurology* 1989;39:1118–1120.

54. Allal J, Thomas Ph, Mazzonelli H. *Borrelia* isolated from cerebrospinal fluid in a French case of Lyme disease. *Ann Rheum Dis* 1986;45:789–790.

55. Steere AC. Lyme disease. *N Engl J Med* 1989;321:586–596.

56. Snydman DR, Schenkein DP, Berardi VP, Lastavica CC, Pariser KM. *Borrelia burgdorferi* in joint fluid in chronic Lyme arthritis. *Ann Intern Med* 1986;104:798–800.

57. Schmidli H, Hunziker T, Moesli P, Schaad UB. Cultivation of *Borrelia burgdorferi* from joint fluid three months after treatment of facial palsy due to Lyme borreliosis. *J Infect Dis* 1988;158:905–906.

58. Johnson YE, Duray PH, Steere AC, et al. Lyme arthritis: Spirochetes found in synovial microangiopathic lesions. *Am J Pathol* 1985;118:26–34.

59. Åsbrink E, Hovmark A. Successful cultivation of spirochetes from skin lesions of patients with erythema chronicum migrans Afzelius and acrodermatitis chronica atrophicans. *APMIS (B)* 1985;93:161–163.

60. Wokke JHJ, de Koning J, Stanek G, Jennekens FGI. Chronic muscle weakness caused by *Borrelia burgdorferi* meningoradiculitis. *Ann Neurol* 1987;22:389–392.

61. Dattwyler RJ, Volkman DJ, Halperin JJ, Luft BJ, Thomas J, Golightly MG. Specific immune responses in Lyme borreliosis: Characterization of T cell and B cell responses to *Borrelia burgdorferi*. *Ann NY Acad Sci* 1988;539:93–102.

62. Dattwyler RJ, Thomas JA, Benach JL, Golightly MG. Cellular immune response in Lyme disease: The response to mitogens, live *Borrelia burgdorferi*, NK cell function and lymphocyte subsets. *Zentralbl Bakteriol Mikrobiol Hyg [A]* 1986;263:151–159.

63. Dattwyler RJ, Volkman DJ, Luft BJ, Halperin JJ, Thomas J, Golightly MG. Seronegative Lyme disease: Dissociation of specific T- and B-lymphocyte responses to *Borrelia burgdorferi*. *N Engl J Med* 1988;319:1441–1446.

64. Sigal LH, Steere AC, Freeman DH, et al. Proliferative responses of mononuclear cells in Lyme disease: Reactivity to *Borrelia burgdorferi* antigens is greater in joint fluid than in blood. *Arthritis Rheum* 1986;29:761–769.

65. Pachner AR, Steere AC, Sigal LH, et al. Antigen-specific proliferation of CSF lymphocytes in Lyme disease. *Neurology* 1985;35:1642–1644.

66. Sigal LH. Lyme disease, 1988: Immunologic manifestations and possible immunopathogenetic mechanisms. *Semin Arthritis Rheum* 1989;18:151–167.

67. Moffat CM, Sigal LH, Steere AC, Freeman DH, Dwyer JM. Cellular immune findings in Lyme disease: Correlation with serum IgM and disease activity. *Am J Med* 1984;77:625–632.

68. Golightly M, Thomas J, Volkman D, Dattwyler R. Modulation of natural killer cell activity by *Borrelia burgdorferi*. *Ann NY Acad Sci* 1988;539:431–433.

69. Thomas JA, Lipschitz R, Golightly MG, Dattwyler RJ. Immunoregulatory abnormalities in *Borrelia burgdorferi* infection. *Ann NY Acad Sci* 1988;539:431–433.

70. Sigal LH, Moffat CM, Steere AC, Dwyer JM. Cellular immune findings in Lyme disease. *Yale J Biol Med* 1984;57:595–598.

71. Shrestha M, Grodzicki RL, Steere AC. Diagnosing early Lyme disease. *Am J Med* 1985;78:235–239.

72. Craft JE, Grodzicki RL, Steere AC. The antibody response in Lyme disease: Evaluation of diagnostic tests. *J Infect Dis* 1984;149:789–795.

73. Craft JE, Fischer DK, Shimamato GT, Steere AC. Antigens of *Borrelia burgdorferi* recognized during Lyme disease: Appearance of a new immunoglobulin M response and expansion of the immunoglobin G response late in the illness. *J Clin Invest* 1986;78:934–939.

74. Magnarelli LA, Anderson JF. Early detection and persistence of antibodies to *Borrelia burgdorferi* in persons with Lyme disease. *Zentralbl Bakteriol Mikrobiol Hyg [A]* 1986;263:393–399.

75. Coleman JL, Benach JL. Isolation of antigenic components from the Lyme disease spirochete: Their role in early activity of skin and joints. *J Infect Dis* 1987;155:756–765.

76. Sigal LH, Steere AC, Dwyer JM. *In vivo* and *in vitro* evidence of B cell hyperactivity during Lyme disease. *J Rheumatol* 1988;15:648–654.

77. Benach JL, Fleit HB, Habicht GS, Coleman JL, Bosler EM, Lane BP. Interactions of phagocytes with the Lyme disease spirochete: Role of the Fc receptor. *J Infect Dis* 1984;150:497–507.

78. Kochi SK, Johnson RC. Role of immunoglobulin G in killing of *Borrelia burgdorferi* by the classical complement pathway. *Infect Immun* 1988;56:314–321.

79. Weber K, Schierz G, Wilske B, et al. Reinfection in erythema migrans disease. *Infection* 1986;14:38–41.

80. Pfister H-W, Neubert U, Wilske B, Preac-Mursic V, Einhäupl KM, Borasio GD. Reinfection with *Borrelia burgdorferi*. *Lancet* 1986;2:984–985.
81. Habicht GS. Lyme disease: Antigens of *Borrelia burgdorferi* and immune responses to them. *Ann NY Acad Sci* 1988;539:112–114.
82. Benach JL, Coleman JL, Garcia-Monco JC, Deponte PC. Biological activity of *Borrelia burgdorferi* antigens. *Ann NY Acad Sci* 1988;539:115–125.
83. Habicht GS, Beck G, Benach JL, Coleman JL. *Borrelia burgdorferi* lipopolysaccharide and its role in the pathogenesis of Lyme disease. *Zentralbl Bakteriol Mikrobiol Hyg [A]* 1986;263: 137–141.
84. Beck G, Habicht GS, Benach JL, Coleman JL, Lysik RM, O'Brien RF. A role for interleukin-1 in the pathogenesis of Lyme disease. *Zentralbl Bakteriol Mikrobiol Hyg [A]* 1986;263:133–136.
85. Habicht GS, Beck G, Benach JL. The role of interleukin-1 in the pathogenesis of Lyme disease. *Ann NY Acad Sci* 1988;439:80–86.
86. Habicht GS, Beck G, Benach JL, Coleman JL, Leichtling KD. Lyme disease spirochetes induce human and murine interleukin 1 production. *J Immunol* 1985;134:3147–3154.
87. Steere AC, Brinckerhoff CE, Miller DJ, Drinker H, Harris ED Jr, Malawista SE. Elevated levels of collagenase and protaglandin E2 from synovium associated with erosion of cartilage and bone in a patient with chronic Lyme arthritis. *Arthritis Rheum* 1980;23:591–599.
88. Steere AC, Pachner AR, Malawista SE. Neurologic abnormalities of Lyme disease: Successful treatment with high-dose intravenous penicillin. *Ann Intern Med* 1983;99:767–772.
89. Ackermann R, Rehse-Küpper B, Gollmer E, Schmidt R. Chronic neurologic manifestations of erythema migrans borreliosis. *Ann NY Acad Sci* 1988;539:16–23.
90. Reik L. *Borrelia burgdorferi* infection: A neurologist's perspective. *Ann NY Acad Sci* 1988;539:1–3.
91. Garcia-Monco JC, Fernandez-Villar B, Benach JL. Adherence of the Lyme disease spirochete to glial cells and cells of glial origin. *J Infect Dis* 1989;160:497–506.
92. Steere AC, Malawista SE, Hardin JA, Ruddy S, Askenase PW, Andiman WA. Erythema chronicum migrans and Lyme arthritis: The enlarging clinical spectrum. *Ann Intern Med* 1977;86:685–698.
93. Reik L, Steere AC, Bartenhagen NH, Shope RE, Malawista SE. Neurologic abnormalities of Lyme disease. *Medicine (Baltimore)* 1979;58:281–294.
94. Schutzer SE, Coyle PK, Belman AL, Golightly MG, Drulle J. Sequestration of antibody to *Borrelia burgdorferi* in immune complexes in seronegative Lyme disease. *Lancet* 1990;1: 312–315.
95. Coyle PK, Schutzer SE. Cerebrospinal fluid immune complexes in Lyme disease. *Ann Neurol* 1988;24:142.
96. Reik L, Smith L, Khan A, Nelson W. Demyelinating encephalopathy in Lyme disease. *Neurology* 1985;32:1302–1305.
97. Kohler H, Kern U, Kasper J, Rehse-Küpper B, Thoden U. Chronic central nervous system involvement in Lyme borreliosis. *Neurology* 1988;38:863–867.
98. Pachner AR. *Borrelia burgdorferi* in the nervous system: The new "great imitator." *Ann NY Acad Sci* 1988;539:56–64.
99. Garcia-Monco JC, Coleman JL, Benach JL. Antibodies to myelin basic protein in Lyme disease. *J Infect Dis* 1988;158:667–668.
100. Baig S, Olsson T, Link H. Predominance of *Borrelia burgdorferi* specific B cells in cerebrospinal fluid in neuroborreliosis. *Lancet* 1989;2:71–74.
101. Martin R, Ortlauf J, Sticht-Groh V, Bogdahn U, Goldmann S, Mertens HG. *Borrelia burgdorferi*-specific and autoreactive T-cell lines from cerebrospinal fluid in Lyme radiculomyelitis. *Ann Neurol* 1988;24:509–516.
102. Aberer E, Brunner C, Suchanek G, et al. Molecular mimicry and Lyme borreliosis: A shared antigenic determinant between *Borrelia burgdorferi* and human tissue. *Ann Neurol* 1989;26:732–737.
103. Sigal LH, Tatum A. Lyme disease patients' serum contains IgM antibodies to *Borrelia burgdorferi* that cross-react with neuronal antigens. *Neurology* 1988;38:1439–1442.
104. Pachner AR, Steere AC. The triad of neurologic manifestations of Lyme disease: Meningitis, cranial neuritis and radiculoneuritis. *Neurology* 1985;35:47–53.
105. Vallat JM, Hugon M, Lubeau M, Leboutet MJ, Dumas M, Desproges-Gotteron R. Tick-bite meningoradiculoneuritis: Clinical, electrophysiologic, and histologic findings in 10 cases. *Neurology* 1987;37:749–753.

106. Halperin JJ, Little BW, Coyle PK, Dattwyler RJ. Lyme disease: Cause of a treatable peripheral neuropathy. *Neurology* 1987;37:1700–1706.
107. Kristoferitsch W, Sluga E, Graf M, et al. Neuropathy associated with acrodermatitis chronica atrophicans: Clinical and morphological features. *Ann NY Acad Sci* 1988;539: 35–45.
108. Lubeau M, Vallat JM, Hugon J, Dumas M, Desproges-Gotteron R. Tick bite meningoradiculitis: Ten cases. *Zentralbl Bakteriol Mikrobiol Hyg [A]* 1986;263:321–323.
109. Sterman AB, Nelson S, Barclay P. Demyelinating neuropathy accompanying Lyme disease. *Neurology* 1982;32:1302–1305.
110. Graf M, Kristoferitsch W, Baumhackl U, Zeitlhofer J. Electrophysiologic findings in meningopolyneuritis of Garin-Bujadoux-Bannwarth. *Zentralbl Bakteriol Mikrobiol Hyg [A]* 1986;263:324–327.
111. Reik L, Burgdorfer W, Donaldson JO. Neurologic abnormalities in Lyme disease without erythema chronicum migrans. *Am J Med* 1986;81:73–78.
112. Ackermann R, Horstrup P, Schmidt R. Tick-borne meningopolyneuritis (Garin-Bujadoux, Bannwarth). *Yale J Biol Med* 1984;57:485–490.
113. Steere AC, Gibofsky A, Patarroyo ME, Winchester RJ, Hardin JA, Malawista SE. Chronic Lyme arthritis: Clinical and immunogenetic differentiation from rheumatoid arthritis. *Ann Intern Med* 1979;90:896–901.
114. Steere AC. Pathogenesis of Lyme arthritis: Implications for rheumatic disease. *Ann NY Acad Sci* 1988;539:87–92.
115. Kristoferitsch W, Mayr WR. HLA-DR in meningopolyneuritis of Garin-Bujadoux-Bannwarth: Contrast to Lyme disease. *J Neurol* 1984;231:271–272.
116. Wokke JHJ, van Doorn PA, Brand A, Schreuder GMT, Vermeulen M. Association of HLA-DR2 antigen with serum IgG antibodies against *Borrelia burgdorferi* in Bannwarth's syndrome. *J Neurol* 1988;235:415–417.
117. Majsky, Bojar M, Jirous J. Lyme disease and HLA-DR antigens. *Tissue Antigens* 1987;30: 188–189.

5

Pathology

General Pathologic Features

The histopathologic picture in Lyme disease reflects the host's immunologic response to the presence of *Borrelia burgdorferi* in its tissues.[1] Typically there is an inflammatory cell infiltrate, often perivascular, comprised mainly of T and B lymphocytes, along with varying numbers of plasma cells, macrophages, dendritic immune cells, and tissue mast cells. Similar changes have been detected in most of the tissues involved clinically, and the causative organism has been demonstrated in virtually all of these except for the peripheral nerves and autonomic ganglia. Tissue necrosis is rare, and giant cells and gummas have not been described so far. In later stages, vascular thickening and, sometimes, occlusion are prominent in some tissues, particularly the skin and joints, but fibrinoid necrosis of vessels and neutrophil fragmentation have not been reported.[1–3]

The earliest histologic change is in the skin at the site of the tick bite where the typical changes of an arthropod bite occur: a central area of ulceration underlain by polymorphonuclear leukocytes (PMNs), macrophages, eosinophils, lymphocytes and mast cells and, sometimes, areas of collagen necrosis and hemorrhage.[2]

Following inoculation by the tick bite, the organisms proliferate locally and spread through the skin, producing the skin lesion, erythema migrans (EM). The spirochetes can be demonstrated histologically at the periphery of the spreading skin lesion,[4–6] and the usual lymphoplasmacytic infiltrate is present around small vessels in the papillary and upper reticular dermis.[1,2,4,6,7] The vascular endothelium may be swollen, and there is an occasional lymphocyte in the endothelial cell cytoplasm, but frank vasculitis is not present.[1,2]

When hematogenous dissemination occurs, multiple secondary skin lesions, containing spirochetes and histologically indistinguishable from the

35

primary EM, often develop.[4] At the same time, spirochetes and round cell infiltrates appear in a number of other organs, particularly those of the reticuloendothelial system.[1-3] Plasma cells proliferate in the paracortical region of the lymph nodes and perivascularly in the spleen and are accompanied by large pleomorphic polyclonal immunoblasts. Lymphoplasmacytic cell infiltrates are also present in the portal triads of the liver, and occasional triad vessels show "changes suggestive of mild vasculitis."[2] Lymphocytic interstitial pneumonitis is also seen at this stage.

In fetal cases the organism is present in brain, meninges, subarachnoid space, myocardium, adrenal gland, and liver, but there are no accompanying inflammatory changes.[8,9]

The heart is involved later, usually after the hyperplasia of the reticuloendothelial system has subsided. Cardiac involvement is characterized by the same infiltration of lymphocytes, plasma cells, and macrophages in all three cardiac layers. The organisms can be visualized extracellularly in the heart, and there is endothelial swelling in and lymphoplasmacytic infiltration around scattered small vessels. In larger vessels, the adventitia also can be infiltrated, sometimes producing an obliterative endarteritis.[2,10,11]

Similar vessel changes are seen in the synovium in Lyme arthritis. In the small arteries in the synovial stroma, there are intimal cell proliferation and varying degrees of collagenization, sometimes with an increase in adventitial cells causing onion skin thickening and luminal obliteration. Spirochetes are present in the synovium and synovial fluid in small numbers, rarely in the vascular endothelium or in a perivascular location. There is, in addition, an increase in the number of synovial cells, infiltration of lymphocytes and plasma cells, aggregation of lymphocytes into follicles, and an increase in the number of mast cells and tissue macrophages, often accompanied by fibrin deposition in the subsynovial stroma.[1,3,12]

Occlusive vascular changes also occur in the skin and subcutaneous tissues in a number of the skin lesions associated with late Lyme disease.[1,2] Similar findings have been described in biopsy specimens from Lyme disease patients with acrodermatitis chronica atrophicans (ACA), eosinophilic fascitis, lichen sclerosus et atrophicus (LSA), ulnar fibrous nodules, and morphea. The vascular changes in the skin are often accompanied by thickening of the dermis by excess collagen, and living spirochetes are still present in these lesions years after the onset: They can be both demonstrated histologically[5] and isolated in culture.[13]

Central Nervous System Pathology

Lymphoplasmacytic infiltration also occurs in the CNS, although less is known about CNS pathology in general because of the small amount of material available. Biopsy specimens and autopsy material from a few fatal cases with early CNS involvement have shown sheet-like round cell infiltration in the meninges and around small vessels in the gray matter closest to the meninges (Figure 5–1).[2] These same vessels have shown endothelial swelling but no true vasculitis. In one autopsy case, these perivascular infiltrates were accompanied by disseminated small foci of necrosis in the cerebrum and brain stem.[14] In two others, perivascular lymphoplasmacytic infiltrates were present in the meninges and spinal cord.[15,16] In a fourth, there was more diffuse infiltration of the spinal cord in addition to the meningeal and perivascular infiltration.[17]

In other cases, brain biopsy specimens have shown less intense, round cell infiltration, and tissue changes have been confined to increases in microglial cells with the formation of glial nodules (Figure 5–2), an increase in astroglia (Figure 5–3), and mild spongiform changes (Figure 5–4).[1,2,18] Spirochetes have been demonstrated within the brain parenchyma in at least two patients, by silver staining in one (Figure 5–5)[18] and by immunohistochemical techniques in the other (Figure 5–6).[19]

To my knowledge, the pathologic changes in patients with late neurologic involvement have not been described.

Peripheral Nervous System Pathology

Slightly more is known about the pathology of peripheral nerves in Lyme disease. Fatal cases have shown perivascular round cell infiltrates in the nerve roots.[15,17] In biopsied sural nerve, similar changes have been described in

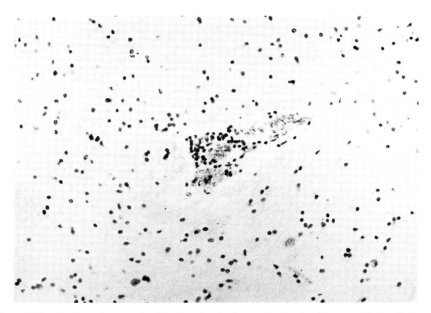

Figure 5–1. Perivascular round cell infiltration in the cerebral cortex from a patient with Lyme disease with encephalitis. (Photograph courtesy of Dr. Paul Duray, Department of Pathology, Fox Chase Cancer Center, Philadelphia, PA.)

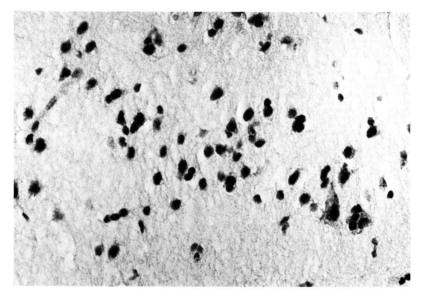

Figure 5–2. Cerebral cortical glial nodule in a patient with Lyme disease with encephalitis. (Photograph courtesy of Dr. Paul Duray, Department of Pathology, Fox Chase Cancer Center, Philadelphia, PA.)

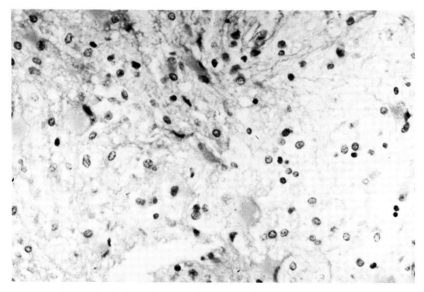

Figure 5–3. Gliosis in the frontal cortex in Lyme encephalitis. (Photograph courtesy of Dr. Paul Duray, Department of Pathology, Fox Chase Cancer Center, Philadelphia, PA.)

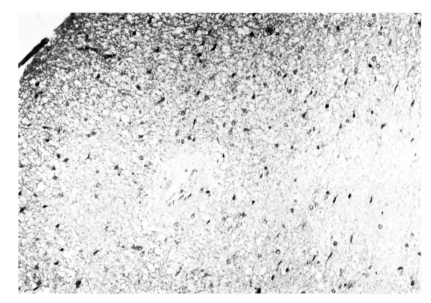

Figure 5–4. Spongiosis in the frontal cortex in Lyme encephalitis. (Photograph courtesy of Dr. Paul Duray, Department of Pathology, Fox Chase Cancer Center, Philadelphia, PA.)

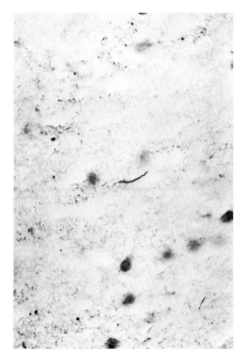

Figure 5–5. *Borrelia burgdorferi* in the cerebral cortex in Lyme encephalitis. Dieterle stain. (Photograph courtesy of Dr. Paul Duray, Department of Pathology, Fox Chase Cancer Center, Philadelphia, PA.)

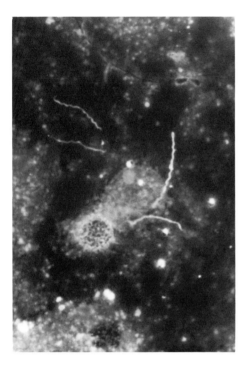

Figure 5–6. *Borrelia burgdorferi* in frontal cortex imprint stained with monoclonal antibody H5332. (Photograph courtesy of Dr. Alan MacDonald, Department of Pathology, Southampton Hospital, Southampton, NY.)

meningopolyneuritis, distal axonopathy of late Lyme disease, and the neuropathy that accompanies ACA.[16,20–25] Typical changes include axonal degeneration, loss of large myelinated fibers (Figure 5–7), epineurial perivascular infiltration of lymphocytes and plasma cells (Figure 5–8), luminal thrombosis, pericapillary plasma cell infiltrates in the perineurium and endoneurium, and infiltration of the interstitium. Segmental demyelination has been observed in only one patient.[22] Spirochetes have not been observed in peripheral nerve, however, and immune complexes, complement, and immunoglobulin have not been seen in biopsy specimens. In one patient, though, IgA and IgM containing plasma cells were present beneath the perineurium.[25] Similar aggregates and groups of lymphocytes can also infiltrate autonomic ganglia and their afferent and efferent rootlets (Figure 5–9).[1,2]

Skeletal Muscle Pathology

A number of cases of inflammatory myopathy in both early and late disseminated Lyme disease have now been reported, several with biopsy confirmation.[26–32] The usual histopathologic finding in early disease has been an interstitial myositis with lymphoplasmacytic infiltration of the perimysium and of the interstitium within the muscle bundles, mainly around small blood vessels.[2,27,29,31] In one additional case, there was a noninflammatory

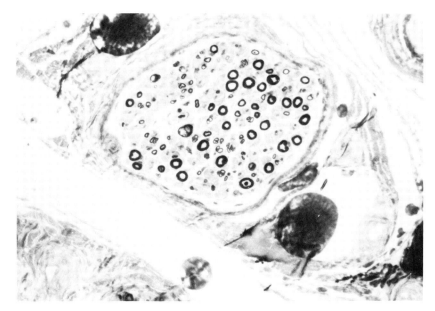

Figure 5–7. Cross section of a sural nerve fascicle from a patient with meningopolyneuritis, showing loss of large myelinated fibers.

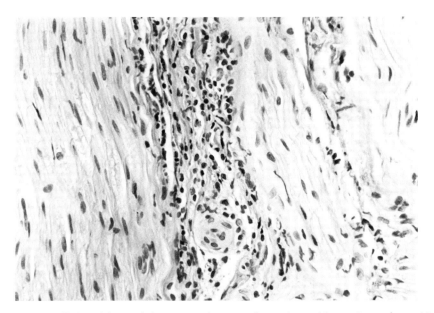

Figure 5–8. Epineurial vessel from a sural nerve of a patient with meningopolyneuritis, showing perivascular round cell infiltration.

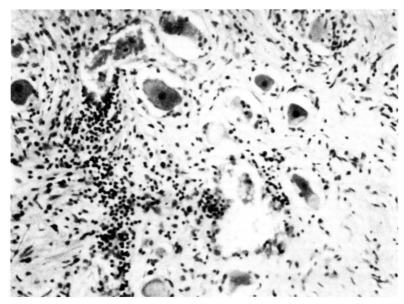

Figure 5–9.   Lymphoplasmacytic infiltration of an autonomic ganglion in a fatal case of Lyme disease. (Photograph courtesy of Dr. Paul Duray, Department of Pathology, Fox Chase Cancer Center, Philadelphia, PA.)

necrotizing myopathy.[28] *B. burgdorferi* has been identified in early cases between muscle fibers, particularly in areas of edema, both by silver staining and by immunogold techniques, but culture attempts have been unsuccessful so far.[2,27,31]

In several patients with ACA, focal nodular myositis with muscle fiber degeneration has been present.[29,31] In these cases, examination of biopsy specimens showed focal perivascular infiltration of histiocytes and lymphocytes with necrosis, phagocytosis, and degeneration of adjacent muscle fibers. Spirochetes were present in the muscle on silver stains.[29] In one other, biopsy specimens showed inclusion body myositis.[31]

References

1. Duray PH, Steere AC. Clinical pathologic correlations of Lyme disease by stage. *Ann NY Acad Sci* 1988;539:65–79.
2. Duray PH. Histopathology of clinical phases of human Lyme disease. *Rheum Dis Clin North Am* 1989;15:691–710.
3. Duray PH. Clinical pathologic correlations of Lyme disease. *Rev Infect Dis* 1989;11(suppl 6):S1487–S1493.
4. Berger BW. Erythema chronicum migrans of Lyme disease. *Arch Dermatol* 1984;120:1017–1021.
5. Frithz A, Lagerholm B. Acrodermatitis chronica atrophicans, erythema chronicum migrans and lymphadenosis benigna cutis—spirochetal diseases? *Acta Derm Venereol (Stockh)* 1983;63:432–436.

6. Berger BW. Dermatologic manifestations of Lyme disease. *Rev Infect Dis* 1989;11(suppl 6):S1475–S1481.
7. Berger BW. Cutaneous manifestations of Lyme borreliosis. *Rheum Dis Clin North Am* 1989;15:627–634.
8. MacDonald AB, Benach JL, Burgdorfer W. Stillbirth following maternal Lyme disease. *NY State J Med* 1987;87:615–616.
9. Weber K, Bratzke H-J, Neubert U, Wilske B, Duray PH. *Borrelia burgdorferi* in a newborn despite oral penicillin for Lyme borreliosis during pregnancy. *Pediatr Infect Dis J* 1988;7:286–289.
10. Reznick JW, Braunstein DB, Walsh RL. Lyme carditis: Electrophysiologic and histopathologic study. *Am J Med* 1986;81:923–927.
11. Marcus LC, Steere AC, Duray PH, Anderson AE, Mahoney EB. Fatal pancarditis in a patient with co-existing Lyme disease and babesiosis. *Ann Intern Med* 1985;103:374–376.
12. Johnson YE, Duray PH, Steere AC, et al. Lyme arthritis: Spirochetes found in synovial microangiopathic lesions. *Am J Pathol* 1985;118:26–34.
13. Åsbrink E, Hovmark A, Hederstedt B. The spirochetal etiology of acrodermatitis chronica atrophicans Herxheimer. *Acta Derm Venereol (Stockh)* 1984;64:506–512.
14. Hänny PE, Häuselmann HJ. Die Lyme-Krankheit aus der Sicht des Neurologen. *Schweiz Med Wochenschr* 1987;117:901–915.
15. Schaltenbrand G. Chronische aseptische Meningitis. *Nervenarzt* 1949;20:433–442.
16. Meurers B, Kohlhepp W, Gold R, Rohrbach E, Mertens HG. Histopathological findings in the central and peripheral nervous systems in neuroborreliosis: A report of three cases. *J Neurol* 1990;237:113–116.
17. Kohlhepp W, Mertens HG, Oschmann P, Rohrbach E. Akute und chronische Erkrankungen bei zeckenvermittelter Borreliose. *Nervenarzt* 1987;58:557–563.
18. Pachner AR, Duray PH, Steere AC. Central nervous system manifestations of Lyme disease. *Arch Neurol* 1989;46:790–795.
19. MacDonald AB, Miranda JM. Concurrent neocortical borreliosis and Alzheimer's disease. *Hum Pathol* 1987;18:759–761.
20. Vallat JM, Hugon J, Lubeau M, Leboutet MJ, Dumas M, Desproges-Gotteron R. Tick-bite meningoradiculoneuritis: Clinical, electrophysiologic, and histologic findings in 10 cases. *Neurology* 1987;37:749–753.
21. Meier C, Grehl H. Vaskulitische Neuropathie bei Garin-Bujadoux-Bannwarth-Syndrom: ein Beitrag zum Verständnis der Pathologie und Pathogenese neurologischer Komplikationen bei Lyme-Borreliose. *Dtsch Med Wochenschr* 1988;113:135–138.
22. Meier C, Grahmann F, Engelmann A, Dumas M. Pathology of peripheral nerve disorders in Lyme borreliosis. Presented at the Fourth International Conference on Lyme Borreliosis; June 18–21, 1990; Stockholm, Sweden.
23. Camponovo F, Meier C. Neuropathy of vasculitic origin in a case of Garin-Boujadoux-Bannwarth syndrome with positive borrelia antibody response. *J Neurol* 1986;233:69–72.
24. Halperin JJ, Little BW, Coyle PK, Dattwyler RJ. Lyme disease: Cause of a treatable peripheral neuropathy. *Neurology* 1987;37:1700–1706.
25. Kristoferitsch W, Sluga E, Graf M, et al. Neuropathy associated with acrodermatitis chronica atrophicans: Clinical and morphological features. *Ann NY Acad Sci* 1988;539:35–45.
26. Kirsch M, Ruben RL, Steere AC, Duray PH, Norden CW, Winkelstein A. Fatal adult respiratory distress syndrome in a patient with Lyme disease. *JAMA* 1988;259:2737–2739.
27. Atlas E, Novak SN, Duray PH, Steere AC. Lyme myositis: Muscle invasion by *Borrelia burgdorferi*. *Ann Intern Med* 1988;109:245–246.
28. Schoenen J, Sianard-Gainko J, Carpentier M, Reznik M. Myositis during *Borrelia burgdorferi* infection (Lyme disease). *J Neurol Neurosurg Psychiatry* 1989;52:1002–1005.
29. Reimers CD, Pongratz DE, Neubert U, et al. Myositis caused by *Borrelia burgdorferi*: Report of four cases. *J Neurol Sci* 1989;91:215–226.
30. DelSette M, Caponnetto C, Fumarola D, Mancardi GL. Unusual neurological manifestations of Lyme disease: A case report. *Ital J Neurol Sci* 1989;10:455–456.
31. Reimers CD, de Koning J, Pilz A, et al. Myositis associated with *Borrelia burgdorferi* infection. Presented at the Fourth International Conference on Lyme Borreliosis; June 18–21, 1990; Stockholm, Sweden.
32. Schmutzhard E, Willeit J, Gerstenbrand F. Meningopolyneuritis Bannwarth with focal nodular myositis: A new aspect in Lyme borreliosis. *Klin Wochenschr* 1986;64:1204–1208.

6

General Clinical Features

The skin, heart, nervous system, and joints are the organ systems most often involved. Because these systems were often involved in sequence in early reports of untreated North American patients, Lyme disease was said to progress in stages: erythema migrans [EM] accompanied by systemic signs and symptoms (stage 1), followed weeks to months later by neurologic or cardiac abnormalities (stage 2), and weeks to years later by arthritis (stage 3).[1] But this classification does not provide for the full spectrum of clinical abnormalities in Lyme disease: Illness can begin in any one of these organ systems, the systems are not always involved sequentially, other skin lesions can develop in later stages, and neurologic abnormalities can accompany arthritis.

While the concept that Lyme disease develops in a series of stages in the typical patient still does provide a useful framework for understanding its clinical features, a modified system of classification proposed by Åsbrink and Hovmark[2] better reflects the pathogenesis of these features and allows for more individual variation (Table 6–1). Under this system, Lyme disease is divided into early and late infection. *Early infection* consists of localized EM (stage 1), often followed within days to weeks by disseminated infection (stage 2). This may be followed in turn, weeks or months later, by intermittent symptoms leading finally to *late* or *persistent infection* (stage 3), defined as beginning a year or more after the initial infection. In an individual patient, any or all stages may be present.

Table 6–1. Major Clinical Manifestations of Lyme Disease by Stage*

Stage	Manifestation
Early	
Localized (stage 1)	Erythema migrans
	Regional adenopathy
	Mild systemic symptoms
Disseminated (stage 2)	Multiple secondary erythema migrans
	Lymphocytoma
	Migratory musculoskeletal pain
	Acute arthritis
	Early neurologic abnormalities[†]
	Generalized adenopathy, splenomegaly
	Carditis
	Severe malaise and fatigue
Late (stage 3)	Acrodermatitis chronica atrophicans
	Chronic arthritis
	Late neurologic abnormalities[‡]
	Chronic fatigue

*Adapted from Steere AC. *N Engl J Med* 1989;321:586–596.
†Lymphocytic meningitis, cranial neuritis, radiculoneuritis, encephalitis, myelitis.
‡Chronic progressive encephalomyelitis, focal encephalitis, mild encephalopathy, distal axonopathy, neuropathy in patients with acrodermatitis.

Early Infection

Localized Infection (Stage 1)

Lyme disease usually begins 3 days to 1 month after a tick bite with the skin lesion EM.[1–9] This begins as a red macule or papule that starts at the site of the bite and expands centrifugally (as *Borrelia burgdorferi* spreads locally in the skin) to form an annular red lesion with central clearing (Color Plate 6–1, page 129). EM develops in about 50% of patients overall (80% in North America and about 40% in Europe) (Figures 6–1 and 6–2) and is the best clinical marker for early disease.[1–9]

The appearance of EM can vary, however.[2,5,7–9] Possible variations include lesions with central ulceration, crusting, or vesiculation; target lesions; erythematous patches with varying intensities of red within the patch but without definite central clearing; triangular and elongated lesions; and lesions with blue shading. The lesions are usually flat, but they can be raised at the center, the edge, or both. The surface is typically smooth, but it can be scaling, and it is often warmer than the surrounding skin. Typical of lesions caused by the bite of crawling arthropods, EM is most often located in the groin or axilla or on the thigh.[1,4,6,9] While the lesion is usually asymptomatic, it may itch or burn in as many as one-third of cases.[2,5,7,8] Accompanying regional adenopathy is common (40%), but constitutional symptoms are

ABNORMALITY

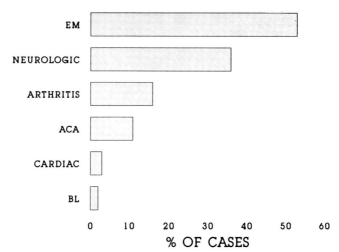

Figure 6–1. Overall worldwide frequency of the major clinical manifestations of Lyme disease. Data compiled from previous studies.[10–28] EM, erythema migrans; ACA, acrodermatitis chronica atrophicans; BL, borrelial lymphocytoma.

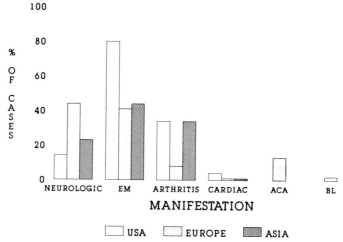

Figure 6–2. Comparative frequency of the major clinical manifestations of Lyme disease among North American, European, and Asian patients. Data compiled from previous studies.[10–28] EM, erythema migrans; ACA, acrodermatitis chronica atrophicans; BL, borrelial lymphocytoma.

usually mild and evanescent.[2–9] Even without treatment, EM usually fades and disappears within 3 or 4 weeks.[1–9]

Disseminated Infection (Stage 2)

Within days or weeks after infection, the spirochete may spread hematogenously to secondary skin sites and to the heart, eye, muscle, bone, joints, reticuloendothelial system, and nervous system.[3]

Multiple secondary annular skin lesions (Color Plate 6–2, page 130) develop in about 25% of North American but fewer European patients.[2–9] They generally spare the palms, soles, and mucous membranes, but not always,[29] and are usually smaller and less migratory than the initial EM.

Involvement of other organ systems leads to an intensification of systemic signs and symptoms.[1,3,4,6] Adenopathy can become generalized, and there may be severe headache accompanied by mild neck stiffness, usually without pleocytosis, both occurring in brief attacks lasting hours. Fever and chills, severe malaise, lethargy, and fatigue are common, as are attacks of migratory musculoskeletal pain centered in the joints, bursae, tendons, muscle, and bone, and lasting hours to days. Other symptoms and signs include cough, splenomegaly, conjunctivitis, and sore throat. Regardless of severity, the signs and symptoms of early dissemination generally last for weeks and then resolve, even without treatment.

Later on during dissemination, weeks or months after illness onset, the organism seems to localize and become sequestered in certain tissues,[3] foremost among them the nervous system. The nervous system is involved in about 40% of untreated patients (15 to 20% of North American and about 50% of European patients) (see Figures 6–1 and 6–2), either while EM is still present or 1 to 6 months later. The typical picture is of a lymphocytic meningitis accompanied by cranial and peripheral neuropathies and radiculopathies that usually last for weeks or months.[30,31]

Cardiac involvement also develops within several weeks of illness onset, affects about 4% of North American and 1% of European patients (see Figure 6–2), and lasts for days to 6 weeks.[3,32–34] Most common is a fluctuating atrioventricular block that can progress to asystole and require a temporary pacemaker, but usually persists for no more than a week. Other less common cardiac abnormalities include diffuse myocarditis, left ventricular dysfunction, fibrinous pericarditis leading to constriction, and fatal pancarditis.[3,32–35]

Localization in the skin at this stage causes another characteristic lesion, borrelial lymphocytoma, lymphocytoma cutis, or lymphadenosis benigna cutis (Color Plate 6–3, page 130),[2,36] especially in Europe where it is present in about 2% of reported cases of Lyme disease (see Figure 6–2). Lymphocytoma is a nodular solitary red or purple lesion containing lymphoid follicles and ranging up to several centimeters in diameter. It is usually located on the nipple in adults or on the earlobe in children, either at the site of the tick bite or remote from it. Borrelial lymphocytoma may occur together with or be preceded by EM, or it can develop as long as 6 to 10 months after the bite and persist for years when untreated. There are often no accompanying systemic symptoms, but some patients with lymphocytoma have regional lymphadenopathy, headache, meningitis, choroiditis, cranial nerve palsies, or arthritis.

Other reported clinical manifestations during this stage of the illness include interstitial pneumonitis,[35,37] hepatitis,[38] necrotizing splenitis,[39] myositis,[40–42] panniculitis,[43] eosinophilic fasciitis,[44] osteomyelitis,[45] choroiditis with retinal detachment,[46] and panophthalmitis.[47]

Somewhat later during dissemination, a mean of 6 months after illness onset (range, 2 weeks to 2 years), about 20% of patients overall (40% of North American and 10% of European patients) (see Figures 6–1 and 6–2) develop arthritis.[1,3,4,48–50] Joint involvement often follows but occasionally precedes stage 2 neurologic abnormalities and is typically a mono- or oligoarticular inflammatory arthritis that occurs in recurrent attacks. One or two large joints, typically the wrist, shoulder, or, especially, the knee, are involved in attacks lasting weeks and sometimes recurring over years. During the attacks, the involved joints are swollen, hot, and painful but not usually red. Accompanying fatigue is common, but other systemic symptoms are usually absent. White blood cell counts in the synovial fluid range between 500 and 100,000 cells/mm^3, mainly polymorphonuclear leukocytes, and the fluid typically contains 3 to 8 g/dL of protein.

Late or Persistent Infection (Stage 3)

In most patients, the attacks of arthritis become less severe and less long lasting during subsequent years, and the number of patients with recurrences decreases by 10 to 20% yearly.[3,48] In some patients, however, the episodes become longer, lasting months rather than weeks, and chronic arthritis (continuous joint inflammation for a year or more), usually of one knee, develops in about 10%.[3,48–50] Chronic arthritis may lead to erosion of cartilage and bone and cause permanent joint disability, but even patients with chronic Lyme arthritis usually improve with time: They rarely have continuous joint inflammation for more than several years.[3,48]

Persistent skin infection is also a feature of late Lyme disease, but, unlike the joint disease, it does not improve spontaneously. The characteristic skin lesion, acrodermatitis chronica atrophicans (ACA),[2,36] is most common in Europe where it is present in as many as 13% of reported cases (see Figure 6–2). ACA is a chronic disorder with long latency and gradual onset. It is rare in childhood, affecting mainly the elderly, particularly women. The lesion begins asymmetrically, usually on the distal parts of the extremities, but occasionally on the trunk. In some patients (18%) it begins on the same extremity where EM was present 6 months to 10 years previously. The first change is a bluish-red discoloration and doughy swelling of the skin that can persist for years, or even decades (Color Plate 6–4, page 130). Eventually, the inflammation is replaced by atrophy of the skin and underlying structures.

Accompanying signs and symptoms include polyneuropathy (40%), local joint deformity (30%), fibrous nodules near the joints, weight loss, fatigue, and personality change.[2] Laboratory abnormalities include hyperglobulinemia, increased erythrocyte sedimentation rate (ESR), and the presence of anti–*B. burgdorferi* antibodies in serum. Examination of skin biopsy specimens confirms the clinical diagnosis: Typical findings are telangiectasia and perivascular lymphoplasmacytic infiltration in the dermis.[2,44]

Other sclerotic skin lesions also may develop during late disease. About 10% of patients with ACA have additional skin lesions that are indistinguishable on clinical and histopathologic grounds from localized scleroderma (morphea) and lichen sclerosus et atrophicus (LSA).[2,35,44] Moreover, other morphea and LSA patients without ACA have had elevated serum titers of anti–*B. burgdorferi* antibodies, and spirochetes have been identified histologically in biopsied skin lesions from 4 of 13 patients with morphea and 6 of 13 with LSA using a specific avidin-biotin-immunoperoxidase technique.[51] In one seropositive patient with morphea, *Borrelia* were cultured from the biopsied lesion.[52] Similarly, elevated antibody titers have been reported in patients with atrophoderma and primary macular atrophy (anetoderma), and anetoderma-like areas of macular atrophy have developed in some patients with ACA.[2] Yet most patients with these skin lesions do not have Lyme disease, and the presence of these lesions, unlike that of EM or ACA, is not diagnostic of *B. burgdorferi* infection.

Persistent and often progressive neurologic abnormalities can similarly develop during late Lyme disease, sometimes after long latency. These abnormalities include chronic progressive encephalomyelitis,[53] focal encephalitis,[54] a mild encephalopathy,[55] distal axonopathy,[56] and an asymmetric polyneuropathy in patients with ACA.[57] These and the other neurologic abnormalities of Lyme disease are described in detail in the chapters that follow.

References

1. Steere AC, Malawista SE, Bartenhagen NH, et al. The clinical spectrum and treatment of Lyme disease. *Yale J Biol Med* 1984;57:453–461.
2. Åsbrink E, Hovmark A. Early and late cutaneous manifestations in *Ixodes*-borne borreliosis (erythema migrans borreliosis, Lyme borreliosis). *Ann NY Acad Sci* 1988;539:4–15.
3. Steere AC. Lyme disease. *N Engl J Med* 1989;321:586–596.
4. Steere AC, Malawista SE, Hardin JA, Ruddy S, Askenase PW, Andiman WA. Erythema chronicum migrans and Lyme arthritis: The enlarging clinical spectrum. *Ann Intern Med* 1977;86:685–698.
5. Berger BW. Erythema chronicum migrans of Lyme disease. *Arch Dermatol* 1984;120:1017–1021.
6. Steere AC, Bartenhagen NH, Craft JE, et al. The early clinical manifestations of Lyme disease. *Ann Intern Med* 1983;99:76–82.
7. Berger BW. Dermatologic manifestations of Lyme disease. *Rev Infect Dis* 1989;11(suppl 6):S1475–S1481.
8. Berger BW. Cutaneous manifestations of Lyme borreliosis. *Rheum Dis Clin North Am* 1989;15:627–633.

9. Åsbrink E. Erythema chronicum migrans Afzelius and acrodermatitis chronica atrophicans: Early and late manifestations of *Ixodes ricinus*-borne *Borrelia* spirochetes. *Acta Derm Venereol Suppl (Stockh)* 1985;118:1–63.

10. Weber K, Puzik A, Becker T. Erythema-migrans Krankheit: Beitrag zur Klinik und Beziehung zur Lyme-Krankheit. *Dtsch Med Wochenschr* 1983;108:1182–1190.

11. Bowen GS, Griffin M, Hayne C, Slade J, Schulze TL, Parkin W. Clinical manifestations and descriptive epidemiology of Lyme disease in New Jersey, 1978 to 1982. *JAMA* 1984;251:2236–2240.

12. Schmidt R, Kabatzki J, Hartung S, Ackermann R. Erythema-migrans-Borreliose in der Bundesrepublik Deutschland: Epidemiologie und klinisches Bild. *Dtsch Med Wochenschr* 1985;110:1803–1807.

13. Aeschlimann A, Chamot E, Gigon F, Jeanneret J-P, Kesseler D, Walther C. *B. burgdorferi* in Switzerland. *Zentralbl Bakteriol Mikrobiol Hyg [A]* 1986;263:450–458.

14. Benach JL, Coleman JL. Clinical and geographic characteristics of Lyme disease in New York. *Zentralbl Bakteriol Mikrobiol Hyg [A]* 1986;263:477–482.

15. Bózsik BP, Lakos A, Budai J, Telegdy L, Ambrózy G. Occurrence of Lyme borreliosis in Hungary. *Zentralbl Bakteriol Mikrobiol Hyg [A]* 1986;263:466–467.

16. Dournon E, Assous M. Lyme disease in France. *Zentralbl Bakteriol Mikrobiol Hyg [A]* 1986;263:464–465.

17. Schmidt R, Kabatzki J, Hartung S, Ackermann R. Erythema chronicum migrans disease in the Federal Republic of Germany. *Zentralbl Bakteriol Mikrobiol Hyg [A]* 1986;263:435–441.

18. Stanek G, Flamm H, Groh V, et al. Epidemiology of *Borrelia* infections in Austria. *Zentralbl Bakteriol Mikrobiol Hyg [A]* 1986;263:442–449.

19. Trevisan G, Crovato F, Marcuccio C, Fumarola D, Scarpa C. Lyme disease in Italy. *Zentralbl Bakteriol Mikrobiol Hyg [A]* 1986;263:459–463.

20. Wilske B, Steinhuber R, Bergmeister H, et al. Lyme-Borreliose in Süddeutschland: epidemiologische Daten zum Auftreten von Erkrankungsfällen sowie zur Durchseuchung von Zecken (*Ixodes ricinus*) mit *Borrelia burgdorferi*. *Dtsch Med Wochenschr* 1987;112:1730–1736.

21. Centers for Disease Control. Lyme disease—Connecticut. *MMWR* 1988;37:1–3.

22. Chengxu A, Yuxin W, Yongguo Z, et al. Clinical manifestations and epidemiological characteristics of Lyme disease in Hailin County, Heilongjiang Province, China. *Ann NY Acad Sci* 1988;539:302–313.

23. Dekonenko EJ, Steere AC, Berardi V, Kravchuk LN. Lyme borreliosis in the Soviet Union: A cooperative US-USSR report. *J Infect Dis* 1988;158:748–753.

24. Stanek G, Pletschette M, Flamm H, et al. European Lyme borreliosis. *Ann NY Acad Sci* 1988;539:274–282.

25. Ciesielski CA, Markowitz LE, Horsley R, Hightower AW, Russell H, Broome CV. Lyme disease surveillance in the United States, 1983–1986. *Rev Infect Dis* 1989;11(suppl 6):S1435–S1441.

26. Lastavica CC, Wilson ML, Berardi VP, Spielman A, Deblinger RD. Rapid emergence of a focal epidemic of Lyme disease in coastal Massachusetts. *N Engl J Med* 1989;320:133–137.

27. Millner M, Schimek MG, Spork D, Schnizer M, Stanek G. Lyme borreliosis in children: A controlled clinical study based on ELISA values. *Eur J Pediatr* 1989;148:527–530.

28. Williams CL, Strobino B, Lee A, et al. Lyme disease in childhood: Clinical and epidemiologic features of ninety cases. *Pediatr Infect Dis J* 1990;9:10–14.

29. Burke WA, Steinbaugh JR, O'Keefe EJ. Lyme disease mimicking secondary syphilis. *J Am Acad Dermatol* 1986;14:137–139.

30. Reik L, Steere AC, Bartenhagen NH, Shope RE, Malawista SE. Neurologic abnormalities of Lyme disease. *Medicine (Baltimore)* 1979;58:281–294.

31. Pachner AR, Steere AC. The triad of neurologic manifestations of Lyme disease: Meningitis, cranial neuritis and radiculoneuritis. *Neurology* 1985;35:47–53.

32. Steere AC, Batsford WP, Weinberg M, et al. Lyme carditis: Cardiac abnormalities of Lyme disease. *Ann Intern Med* 1980;93:8–16.

33. Reznick JW, Braunstein DB, Walsh RL. Lyme carditis: Electrophysiologic and histopathologic study. *Am J Med* 1986;81:923–927.

34. van der Linde MR. Lyme carditis: Clinical characteristics of 105 documented cases. Presented at the Fourth International Conference on Lyme Borreliosis; June 18–21, 1990; Stockholm, Sweden.

35. Duray PH, Steere AC. Clinical pathologic correlations of Lyme disease by stage. *Ann NY Acad Sci* 1988;539:65–79.

36. Weber K, Schierz G, Wilske B, Preac-Mursik V. European erythema migrans disease and related disorders. *Yale J Biol Med* 1984;57:463–471.
37. Kirsch M, Ruben FL, Steere AC, Duray PH, Norden CW, Winkelstein A. Fatal adult respiratory distress syndrome in a patient with Lyme disease. *JAMA* 1988;259:2737–2739.
38. Goellner MH, Agger WA, Burgess JH, Duray PH. Hepatitis due to recurrent Lyme disease. *Ann Intern Med* 1988;108:707–708.
39. Rank EL, Dias SM, Hasson J, et al. Human necrotizing splenitis caused by *Borrelia burgdorferi*. *Am J Clin Pathol* 1989;91:493–498.
40. Reimers CD, Pongratz DE, Neubert U, et al. Myositis caused by *Borrelia burgdorferi*: Report of four cases. *J Neurol Sci* 1989;91:215–226.
41. Reimers CD, de Koning J, Pilz A, et al. Myositis associated with *Borrelia burgdorferi* infection. Presented at the Fourth International Conference on Lyme Borreliosis; June 18–21, 1990; Stockholm, Sweden.
42. Atlas E, Novak SN, Duray PH, Steere AC. Lyme myositis: Muscle invasion by *Borrelia burgdorferi*. *Ann Intern Med* 1988;109:245–246.
43. Kramer N, Rickert RR, Brodkin RH, Rosenstein ED. Septal panniculitis as a manifestation of Lyme disease. *Am J Med* 1986;81:149–152.
44. Duray PH. Histopathology of clinical phases of human Lyme disease. *Rheum Dis Clin North Am* 1989;15:691–710.
45. Jacobs JC, Stevens M, Duray PH. Lyme disease simulating septic arthritis. *JAMA* 1986;256:1138–1139.
46. Bialasiewicz AA, Ruprecht KW, Naumann GO, Blenk H. Bilateral diffuse choroiditis and exudative retinal detachments with evidence of Lyme disease. *Am J Ophthalmol* 1988;105:419–420.
47. Steere AC, Duray PH, Kauffmann DJH, Wormser GP. Unilateral blindness caused by infection with the Lyme disease spirochete, *Borrelia burgdorferi*. *Ann Intern Med* 1985;103:382–384.
48. Steere AC, Schoen RT, Taylor E. The clinical evolution of Lyme arthritis. *Ann Intern Med* 1987;107:725–731.
49. Lawson JP, Steere AC. Lyme arthritis: Radiologic findings. *Radiology* 1985;154:37–43.
50. Steere AC, Gibofsky A, Patarroyo ME, Winchester RJ, Hardin JA, Malawista SE. Chronic Lyme arthritis: Clinical and immunogenetic differentiation from rheumatoid arthritis. *Ann Intern Med* 1979;90:896–901.
51. Aberer E, Stanek G. Histological evidence for spirochetal origin of morphea and lichen sclerosus et atrophicans. *Am J Dermatopathol* 1987;9:374–379.
52. Aberer E, Kollegger H, Kristoferitsch W, Stanek G. Neuroborreliosis in morphea and lichen sclerosus et atrophicus. *J Am Acad Dermatol* 1988;19:820–825.
53. Ackermann R, Rehse-Küpper B, Gollmer E, Schmidt R. Chronic neurologic manifestations of erythema migrans borreliosis. *Ann NY Acad Sci* 1988;539:16–23.
54. Broderick JP, Sandok BA, Mertz LE. Focal encephalitis in a young woman 6 years after the onset of Lyme disease: Tertiary Lyme disease? *Mayo Clin Proc* 1987;62:313–316.
55. Halperin JJ, Pass HL, Anand AK, Luft BJ, Volkman DJ, Dattwyler RJ. Nervous system abnormalities in Lyme disease. *Ann NY Acad Sci* 1988;539:24–34.
56. Halperin JJ, Little BW, Coyle PK, Dattwyler RJ. Lyme disease: Cause of a treatable peripheral neuropathy. *Neurology* 1987;37:1700–1706.
57. Kristoferitsch W, Sluga E, Graf M, et al. Neuropathy associated with acrodermatitis chronica atrophicans: Clinical and morphological features. *Ann NY Acad Sci* 1988;539:35–45.

7

Neurologic Abnormalities in Early Lyme Disease

Symptomatic neurologic involvement develops during early Lyme disease in about 20% of North American and as many as 50% of European patients (see Figure 6–2), at times soon after illness onset. *Borrelia burgdorferi* has been cultured from CSF obtained as early as 18 days after a tick bite,[1] and neurologic symptoms can begin while erythema migrans (EM) is still present: Patients with EM often have headache, neck stiffness, lethargy, or even mild encephalopathy along with their other systemic symptoms, particularly if there are multiple secondary skin lesions.[2–6] The CSF usually is said to be normal in such patients, but in one recent study, 6 of 24 patients with localized EM examined prospectively had a pleocytosis.[7]

Nevertheless, neurologic signs and symptoms develop most commonly during early disseminated (stage 2) infection, weeks to months after illness onset, usually after EM has faded. Then the most common neurologic abnormalities are lymphocytic meningitis, with or without accompanying CNS parenchymal involvement, radicular pains, and cranial and peripheral neuropathies (meningopolyneuritis or Bannwarth's syndrome).[a]

In the typical case (Figure 7–1), neurologic symptoms begin 2 days to 5 months (usually 2 to 4 weeks) after an EM (present in 40 to 50% of patients

---

[a]Unless otherwise noted, the statements in this chapter regarding patients with stage 2 neurologic abnormalities are based on a compilation of data from previous reports[8–93] which contain 1439 cases of early Lyme disease with neurologic involvement from Algeria, Austria, Belgium, Czechoslovakia, Denmark, Germany, France, Ireland, Italy, the Netherlands, Norway, Sweden, Switzerland, the United Kingdom, the United States, and the USSR.

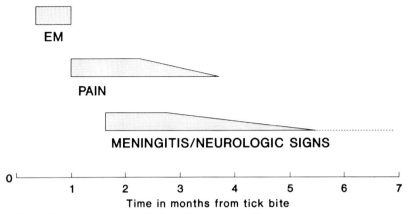

Figure 7–1. Time course of untreated meningopolyneuritis.

overall but as many as 80% of North Americans). About 40% of patients recall an antecedent tick or other insect (4%) bite, the interval between bite and EM usually being 1 to 2 weeks (range, 1 day to 5 months) when both are present. Neurologic symptoms can begin in any month, but they usually do so in summer, particularly July and August. When neurologic symptoms do begin, they are accompanied by systemic signs and symptoms typical of early disseminated disease in up to two-thirds of cases. These include headache, fatigue, fever, myalgia, neck stiffness, nausea and vomiting, arthralgia, photophobia, and acute arthritis, in decreasing order of frequency (Figure 7–2).

Peripheral Nervous System Abnormalities

Involvement of the peripheral nervous system usually begins (in 75 to 80% of cases) with severe radicular pains, paresthesias, or hyperesthesias typically starting 6 weeks after a tick bite or a month after the appearance of EM (range: a few days to 3 months). These begin most often on the trunk or proximal part of the limbs—in some European, but not North American, patients, in the area of the initiating tick bite.[13,25,56,63,85,94] The pains are boring, biting, or tearing in quality; begin acutely or subacutely; and reach a maximum within hours to a few days. There is almost always accompanying nonradicular pain that is more diffuse; tends to localize under the scapulae or over the spine in the low or mid back or neck; is migratory; and is described as burning, gnawing, or tearing in quality. Both the spine and radicular pain tend to be worse at night[13,32,34,84,85,87,92,95] and relatively resistant to analgesics. Once established, the pain can last for months during which it can either remain localized to the original area, spread to additional areas, or move completely

SIGNS AND SYMPTOMS

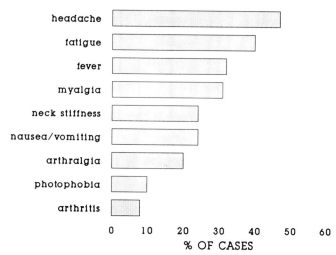

Figure 7–2.   Systemic signs and symptoms present at the onset of neurologic abnormalities in stage 2 Lyme disease.

to new areas. Eventually (within 6 weeks to 3 months) it subsides completely, even without treatment (see Figure 7–1).

Radiculoneuritis

About 75% of patients with pain develop radiculoneuritis, usually within 1 to 4 weeks of its onset (range, a few days to 3 months), or 4 to 8 weeks after EM (see Figure 7–1). Radiculoneuritis occurs in about 40% of patients with stage 2 neurologic abnormalities overall (Figure 7–3), the reported frequency ranging from 30 to 50% in North America[59,60,65,66] to as high as 96% in Europe.[8] Peripheral neuropathy appears to be less common among children with Lyme disease, however, at least in Europe.[19,40,63] When it does occur, radiculoneuritis is almost always accompanied by pleocytosis (in 95% of patients). Accompanying cranial neuropathy is also common (55%), but meningeal symptoms are less frequent (25%).

MOTOR WEAKNESS

Motor weakness begins gradually and can progress over days to weeks as separate extremities are involved in turn. It can advance quickly to atrophy.[13,22,28,34,36,59,65,77,84] The weakness is typically asymmetric and focal or multifocal; it involves the legs twice as often as the arms and, in a number of European patients, has been confined to or is more severe in the limb that was the site of the initial tick bite or EM.[34,83,89] Individual nerves, nerve roots, and plexuses can all be involved; the most common clinical patterns are brachial and lumbosacral plexitis, mononeuritis simplex and multiplex, and motor

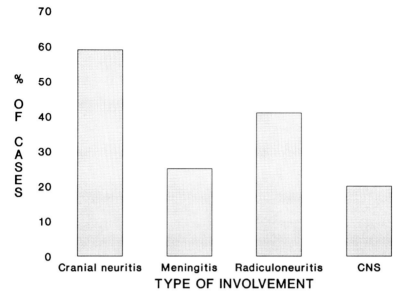

Figure 7–3.   Frequency of major types of neurologic abnormalities in patients with stage 2 Lyme disease involving the nervous system.

radiculitis in the extremities. Distal symmetric polyneuritis is much less common (< 1%).

Yet, in many patients, tendon reflexes are depressed in limbs with normal strength and sensation, suggesting that a more widespread and symmetric but subclinical neuropathy does occur. Tetraparesis can occur in meningopolyneuritis, and at least four cases of a Guillain-Barré–like syndrome in patients with Lyme disease have been reported in detail. In one of these, the clinical picture, CSF findings, and electrophysiologic abnormalities were typical of the Guillain-Barré syndrome (GBS); anti–*B. burgdorferi* antibodies were present in serum and CSF; and the patient improved clinically with antibiotic therapy and plasmapheresis.[96] In two others, the clinical picture was typical of GBS, but there was an accompanying pleocytosis (93 and 35 to 122 cells/mm^3).[52,80] In the fourth, albuminocytologic dissociation was present, but the weakness was asymmetric and there were diffuse denervation potentials, suggesting instead a confluent mononeuritis multiplex.[97] In addition, two further cases of GBS in Lyme disease were reported by Christen et al. but were not described in detail.[98] Finally, in at least five other typical patients with the syndrome, serum but not CSF antibodies to *B. burgdorferi* were present and, in two, they disappeared after antibiotic treatment.[99–101] Whether these cases represent a direct causal relationship between *B. burgdorferi* infection and the GBS rather than a nonspecific triggering effect of the infection, or even a chance association between seropositivity and the neuropathy, is not clear, however.

Other less frequent patterns of motor weakness can also occur. These include motor neuropathy without pleocytosis (10%), motor weakness without preceding pain (10%), paralysis of the diaphragm,[53,63] the cauda equina syndrome,[87] and paralysis of the abdominal wall muscles.[21,63] Sensory symptoms and radicular pains also affect the chest, occurring there 40% as often as in the limbs, but how often intercostal motor neuropathy or thoracic motor radiculopathy occurs is not known as they have not been sought systematically through appropriate electrophysiologic testing, even in patients with thoracic sensory loss.

SENSORY LOSS

Sensory and motor symptoms are equally frequent in patients with radiculoneuritis, but actual sensory loss is less common than motor weakness, occurring in at most 35% of patients with stage 2 neurologic involvement, and probably fewer. When sensory loss does occur, it usually accompanies weakness: Isolated sensory loss develops in only about 5% of patients. The pattern of sensory loss is usually dermatomal, and it may be located anywhere, although lower cervical and thoracic dermatomes, especially those between T-8 and T-12, are involved most often. As with motor weakness, intense radicular pain comes first and is followed by dermatomal hypoesthesia or hyperesthesia, involving 1 or 2 segments, 1 to 4 weeks later (range, a few days to 3 months). Less often, superficial sensation is lost in a nerve pattern in a paretic limb or distally and symmetrically, usually in the lower extremities.

The outcome is usually favorable. Both sensory loss and motor weakness, even in patients with atrophy, typically resolve spontaneously (see Figure 7–1). Strength commonly returns to normal within 2 months, although recovery occasionally takes longer or is incomplete. Sensory loss also usually resolves completely within 1 to 2 months: Residual hypoesthesia is rare.

ELECTROPHYSIOLOGY

Electrophysiologic testing usually points to axonal degeneration in distal nerves as well as nerve roots.[21,25,29,34,36,38,60,68,85] The electroneurographic abnormalities most commonly reported are: slight prolongation of distal motor latencies with normal or only slightly slowed motor nerve conduction velocities (NCVs), decreased amplitude of sensory potentials with slightly slowed sensory NCVs, and decreased amplitude of compound action potentials. Accompanying electromyographic abnormalities include neurogenic interference patterns and denervation potentials in nerve or root distribution. Changes indicating demyelination are less common, but, in occasional patients with radiculoneuritis, denervation potentials are absent, and the motor NCVs are slowed to the 20 to 30 m/sec range.[29,60,80,96] Additional less common abnormalities include slowing of motor NCV in the median nerve in the carpal tunnel and of the ulnar nerve at the elbow.[29] F wave latencies are prolonged in about half of the patients tested.[25,36,80,85] As with the changes in deep tendon reflexes, the electrophysiologic abnormalities are often more widespread than the clinical abnormalities.

Cranial Neuropathies

Cranial neuropathies develop overall in about 60% of patients with stage 2 neurologic involvement (see Figure 7–3), typically about 3 weeks (range, 1 to 270 days) after the onset of EM (in the 40 to 50% of patients in whom EM is present). In some patients, cranial nerve involvement begins while the skin lesion and its associated symptoms are still present, or, more rarely, even before EM appears. There is almost always an accompanying pleocytosis (93%), usually asymptomatic, and concurrent radiculoneuritis is common (45%). Multiple cranial neuropathies are also common, and involvement of each of the cranial nerves except the first has been reported.

NERVE VII

Facial palsy is most common (Figure 7–4). It accounts for 70 to 80% of all cranial nerve palsies in stage 2 and developed in 10% of all patients with Lyme disease in one large series of almost a thousand patients.[18] Both children and adults are affected.

The evolution and outcome of facial palsy are typical of cranial neuropathies in early Lyme disease in general. The weakness begins acutely, usually during the summer months, characteristically developing over 1 or 2 days. When there has been a preceding tick bite or EM on the face or neck, the subsequent facial paralysis is usually on the same side.[20,40,51] Accompanying

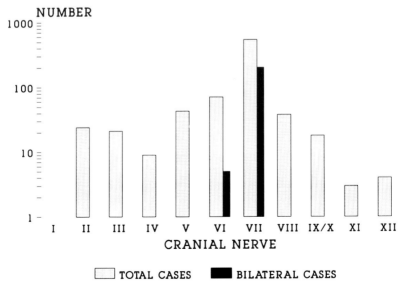

Figure 7–4. Nerves involved in 821 patients with cranial neuropathies during stage 2 Lyme disease.

ipsilateral facial numbness or tingling or ear or jaw pain or both are common. In about 35% of cases, both facial nerves are affected, the two sides becoming paralyzed within a few days to 3 weeks of each other. Topographic localization has been performed infrequently, but loss of taste, hyperacusis, and decreased lacrimation have been reported in some, but not all patients, suggesting that the nerve can be involved at any point along its length. Paralysis is complete in about 60% of cases.[18] Regardless of the degree of paralysis, the outcome is usually favorable with complete recovery within 1 or 2 months, but recovery in some patients may take longer (up to a year) or be incomplete, and permanent facial weakness and hemifacial spasm have been reported in up to 10% of patients.

Facial palsy can be the presenting feature of Lyme disease as it can occur without other accompanying systemic or neurologic signs or symptoms and without antecedent EM.[9,20,39,40,51,58,98,102–105] Then confusion with idiopathic Bell's palsy is likely.

Among unselected patients presenting with facial palsy, the frequency of *B. burgdorferi* infection has varied, depending on the country of origin and the local abundance of ticks. In Sweden, the frequency has varied from 0% in the north,[106] where *Ixodes ricinus* is uncommon, to 20 to 25% in the southeast,[9,58,103,105] where the tick is common. Among Swedish cases from the Stockholm area with onset in summer, the frequency rises to 45% and it reaches 67% in children under age 15 from the same area.[58] Lyme disease is also a common cause of facial palsy in unselected patients from other high incidence areas for Lyme disease in the United States (27%),[104] Austria (40%),[76] and Lower Saxony (60% of children).[20] In the Netherlands, where Lyme disease is less common, on the other hand, no cases of borrelial infection were identified among 69 consecutive cases of facial palsy.[107]

Distinguishing isolated facial palsy due to Lyme disease from Bell's palsy is usually straightforward. Clues to the diagnosis include onset in summer in an area endemic for Lyme disease, history of tick bite or EM, bilateral involvement, and the presence of a lymphocytic pleocytosis and other typical CSF changes.[9,18,20,58,98,102] At the time of the first visit, specific antibody to *B. burgdorferi* is usually present in the serum and, often, in the CSF of patients with facial palsy due to Lyme disease.[9,58,98,102] In occasional patients, serum antibody titers only become elevated 4 to 6 weeks later, so repeated testing is warranted.[58,104]

Electrophysiologic testing of Lyme disease patients with facial palsy has usually shown decreased compound action potentials and denervation of facial muscles, suggesting axonal injury.[36,68,85] In a few patients, however, distal facial nerve motor latencies as much as four to seven times normal have been recorded, a finding more consistent with demyelination.[93]

OTHER CRANIAL NEUROPATHIES

Nerve II. Optic nerve abnormalities make up about 3% of the cranial neuropathies in stage 2. They usually occur in patients with other neurologic deficits. Optic disc edema is most common.[8,63,65,66,93,108–110] In some patients, the papilledema is due to increased intracranial pressure (ICP)[65,108,110] and is accompanied by blind spot enlargement and inferonasal visual field loss.[110] But in others, the ICP is normal[65,109] and the swelling probably represents optic perineuritis caused by extension of inflammation along the meninges of the optic nerves.[110] In still others, there has been sudden visual loss developing over hours or a few days,[73,111,112] suggesting optic neuritis or, in at least one case, ischemic optic neuropathy.[73] Recovery from optic nerve involvement is often incomplete, and permanent visual loss and field defects, residual optic atrophy, and afferent pupillary defects are common, especially when antibiotic therapy is delayed.[48,66,73,83,109,111–113]

Nerves III, IV, and VI. Abnormalities of the nerves innervating the extraocular muscles are relatively common in stage 2 Lyme disease (13% of cranial neuropathies). Abducens palsy is most common (9%),[b] presumably because the sixth nerve is most easily damaged by increased ICP and because its longer course provides more opportunity for injury. Sixth nerve palsy is bilateral about a tenth of the time (see Figure 7–4).[33,64,75,92,93] Paralysis of the third nerve is next most frequent (3%),[c] while involvement of the fourth is uncommon (1%).[8,31,66,77,82,90] Diplopia is the only symptom: Its onset is generally acute or subacute over hours to a day or two. Recovery is usually complete with or without treatment.

Nerve V. Involvement of the trigeminal nerve, typically sensory, accounts for about 6% of cranial neuropathies.[d] Facial paresthesias, numbness, and pain are the usual symptoms. The pain is characteristically neuropathic and burning; in occasional patients, it is more paroxysmal and resembles the pain of trigeminal neuralgia. Sensory signs are less frequent, although some patients do have demonstrable facial sensory loss. The corneal reflex is normally unaffected. Facial sensory abnormalities usually improve spontaneously within weeks to months.

Nerve VIII. Both hearing loss and vertigo can occur in early disseminated Lyme disease and improve following antibiotic therapy, although permanent hearing loss has been reported. While eighth nerve involvement accounted for only 5% of all cranial neuropathies in the series reviewed,[e] recent reports suggest that abnormalities of both the auditory and vestibular systems are more common in early Lyme disease than has been appreciated.[30,46,69] It is not clear whether these abnormalities result mainly from the eighth nerve or from brain stem disease or both, however.

[b]References 8, 12, 31–33, 35, 43, 44, 55, 59, 60, 62–66, 68, 72, 75–77, 81, 83, 90–93.

[c]References 8, 25, 40, 44, 65, 66, 72, 76, 77, 81, 82, 85, 86, 90, 93.

[d]References 8, 12, 31, 44, 48, 63, 65, 72, 75, 76, 83, 90.

[e]References 8, 12, 31, 32, 43, 48, 55, 65, 66, 68, 72, 75, 76, 81, 82, 90, 91.

In one study of 98 consecutive Swedish patients with hearing loss, Hanner et al[30] found serologic evidence for *B. burgdorferi* infection in 17, 15 of whom also had vertigo, and 3 of whom also had facial palsy. All 17 were treated with intravenous penicillin: Hearing improved in 5, one of them after 2 years of hearing loss, and vertigo in 9. A variety of audiometric patterns were seen and included low frequency loss in 9, 6 of whom had a Menière's-type syndrome and 2 of whom had sudden hearing loss; sudden high frequency loss in 4; loss of speech frequencies in 2; and a flat type curve in 1. Most of the lesions were peripheral in type, but brain stem auditory-evoked responses (BAERs) did indicate a retrocochlear or brain stem abnormality in 4 (30%) of 13.

In a second study,[69] the same Swedish investigators examined 73 consecutive patients with vertigo and found 10 (14%) with serum antibodies to *B. burgdorferi,* all of whom had severe, incapacitating vertigo and 4 of whom had associated sensorineural hearing loss. Four of them had attacks of paroxysmal positional vertigo, 4 had attacks of nonpositional vertigo suggestive of Menière's syndrome, and 2 had constant diffuse dizziness and dysequilibrium. Otoneurologic testing revealed evidence for both peripheral and central vestibular lesions. The abnormalities included spontaneous nystagmus in 5, positional nystagmus on electronystagmography in all (paroxysmal and peripheral in 5 and direction changing and presumably central in 5), unilateral caloric unresponsiveness in 5, and abnormal oculomotor tests in 5. BAERs were normal in all 9 patients tested.

In a report from Czechoslovakia of patients with more severe nervous system Lyme disease, however, Krejcova et al[46] concluded that vestibular abnormalities were mostly central in type while auditory abnormalities were both cochlear and brain stem in origin. They found neuro-otologic symptoms in 16 of 39 patients with Lyme disease. Four of the 16 had concomitant radiculoneuritis; 6, encephalomyeloradiculitis; 3, encephalitis; and 1, cranial polyneuritis. Vestibular abnormalities, present in 13 patients, were central in type in 12 and peripheral in 1. These included vertigo in 6, nystagmus (spontaneous in 2, gaze in 3, and positional in 1) in 6, vestibular areflexia in 4, directional preponderance of central origin in 5, impaired optokinetic responses in 3, abnormal saccades in 7, impaired eye tracking movements in 6, and abnormal fixation-suppression tests in 5. Auditory abnormalities were present in 7 cases; symmetric bilateral hearing loss in 4, asymmetric hearing loss in 1, and abnormal BAERs in 5 (prolonged latency of waves III to V and asymmetry of amplitudes). Both the hearing loss and BAER abnormalities resolved within several months.

Nerves IX to XII. Abnormalities of the lower cranial nerves are least common: Together they make up only 3% of all cranial neuropathies. Nerves IX and X[f] are involved more than twice as often as XI and XII.[8,63,72,84,90] Although

---

[f]References 8, 25, 43, 44, 60, 63, 75, 90, 93.

isolated paralysis of the recurrent laryngeal nerve has been attributed to Lyme disease,[114] lower cranial nerve deficits in early Lyme disease usually occur along with other neurologic abnormalities, particularly other cranial neuropathies or radiculoneuropathies. Spontaneous recovery is likely within a few months of onset.

Central Nervous System Abnormalities

Meningitis

Meningitis is the most common neurologic abnormality in stage 2. It may be the presenting feature of Lyme disease as it is preceded by EM in only about 40% of patients overall. When meningitis does follow EM, it usually does so by 2 to 10 weeks.

Eighty to 90% of patients with stage 2 neurologic involvement have pleocytosis, yet only 25% are reported to have meningitis clinically (see Figure 7–3). The true frequency of clinical meningitis may have been underestimated though. It is not always clear from published reports how carefully meningeal symptoms have been sought, and the percentage of symptomatic patients among those with pleocytosis has been quite variable, varying particularly according to the country of origin. When the presence or absence of meningeal symptoms in patients with pleocytosis has been indicated clearly, clinical meningitis has been more common among North American (85%)[60,65] and Swedish (60%)[81,83] patients with pleocytosis than among Austrian (40%)[12,55,75] and German (30%)[8,19,20,37,44,62,63] patients. Children are more likely to be symptomatic than adults.[19,63]

Headache is the most common symptom, affecting 50% (range, 30 to 90%) of patients with CSF inflammation. The pain is usually frontal or occipital and ranges from mild to disabling in intensity. Accompanying mild neck stiffness, usually only on extreme flexion, is present in 20 to 30% of cases. Kernig and Brudzinski signs are rare. Photophobia is present in about 10%, nausea and vomiting in about 25%, and low-grade fever (37.5 to 38.5°C) in 30%.

Symptoms usually begin acutely, persist for 1 or 2 months, then resolve gradually over weeks in untreated patients (see Figure 7–1). But they can be extremely long lasting, particularly in North American patients who sometimes experience fluctuating meningeal symptoms for a year or more (up to 88 weeks).[59,60,65,66,79] During this time, typical patients have repeated attacks of disabling meningeal symptoms lasting weeks alternating with similar several-week periods of milder symptoms. Rarely, the attacks occur at long intervals and are separated by asymptomatic intervals; then recurrent meningitis is simulated.[115]

Patients with meningeal symptoms during stage 2 Lyme disease often have other neurologic abnormalities, particularly facial palsy, but meningitis can occur alone. Then Lyme disease has to be differentiated from other causes of lymphocytic meningitis. Although it is not known how often Lyme disease is the cause in unselected cases of aseptic meningitis from endemic areas, it may be very often: In one report from Germany, 7 of 17 children presenting with aseptic meningitis had serologic or cultural evidence for *B. burgdorferi* infection,[55] and, in another, 41 (16%) of 256 children with aseptic meningitis had specific IgM anti–*B. burgdorferi* antibody in the CSF.[98]

Cerebrospinal Fluid

The CSF pressure may be increased (up to > 500 mm CSF), but it is usually normal.

The fluid typically contains 100 to 200 cells/mm,[3] mainly lymphocytes (Table 7–1). Plasma cells are also common and may make up as much as 25% of the total (average, 9%), particularly during the first few weeks of symptoms.[33,84,95,116–119] Mature plasma cells, plasmacytes with Russell bodies, binucleate plasma cells, and plasma cells undergoing mitosis may all be present.[116,117] CSF cytology may also reveal immunoblasts and foamy macrophages.[116] In occasional patients, prominent immunoblasts, cellular atypia, and mitoses may suggest lymphoreticular malignancy, but the cells can be shown by immunofluorescence to be polyclonal in origin.[116,120] After the first few weeks, plasma cells generally disappear and are replaced by mononuclear cells and histiocytes.[33,95] In rare cases, polymorphonuclear leukocytes (PMNs) predominate at the outset and purulent meningitis is simulated.[15]

The CSF glucose concentration is less than two-thirds the serum glucose concentration in about one-third of patients. The decrease in serum glucose is usually only mild in degree, but values as low as 12 mg/dL have been reported occasionally.[55]

An increase in CSF protein content is also usual, typically in the range of 100 to 300 mg/dL. The increase in protein reflects both barrier leakage and intrathecal synthesis of immunoglobulin: CSF albumin and gamma globulin are both increased. Oligoclonal bands of immunoglobulin are present in 80 to 90% of patients and can be shown to contain both IgG and IgM anti–*B. burgdorferi* antibodies.[121–124] The CSF IgA index is increased in 75%; IgG, in 90%; and IgM, in 90%.[117–119,125–127] Specific anti–*B. burgdorferi* antibody is present in 75 to 100% of patients,[g] depending on the disease duration: Elevated protein, decreased glucose, immunoglobulin abnormalities, and intrathecal antibody synthesis are all more common in cases of longer duration (> 3 weeks).[83,118,122]

Eventually, the CSF abnormalities subside without treatment, usually after clinical recovery has taken place. In the typical patient, the cell count is maximum 3 weeks after meningeal symptoms begin, but it can peak later (up

---

[g]References 20, 25, 32, 40, 58, 62, 76, 77, 83.

Table 7–1.   CFS Findings in Stage 2 Neurologic Lyme Disease

Cell count	5–4000/mm^3 (usually 100–200)
Lymphocytes (%)	> 90% in 75% of patients
Plasma cells (%)	Up to 25% (average, 9%)
Glucose	< 2/3 serum glucose in 35%
Protein	up to 1300 mg/dL (usually 100–300)
Oligoclonal bands	Present in 80–90% of patients
Increase in	
IgA	Present in 75% of patients
IgG	Present in 90% of patients
IgM	Present in 90% of patients
Specific antibody	Present in 75–100% of patients

to 8 weeks), and it commonly remains elevated for 3 to 4 months or more.[33,95,117] The CSF protein concentration normalizes more slowly than the cell count: The protein is often still mildly elevated at 5 to 6 months, but it is generally normal thereafter.[33,95] Immunoglobulin abnormalities are even more long lasting: Oligoclonal bands, increased IgG and IgM, and intrathecal production of specific antibody can persist for years in the absence of clinical signs of disease.[48]

Parenchymal Abnormalities

Cerebral symptoms accompany meningitis in as many as 50% of North American patients with pleocytosis during stage 2, cerebral involvement being apparently more common in those whose meningeal symptoms are more severe.[60,65,66] The symptoms are generally mild and include somnolence, emotional lability, depression, impaired memory and concentration, and behavioral change. In untreated patients, these symptoms tend to fluctuate in intensity for weeks to months before resolving, sometimes in concert with the meningeal symptoms and sometimes independent of them. Cerebral symptoms of this type appear to be less common among European patients with stage 2 involvement, no more than 20% of whom have these mild mental changes,[8,20,63] but cerebral symptoms may have been sought less systematically. Both European and North American patients with such cerebral symptoms usually have abnormal electroencephalograms (EEGs), however, as do some others who appear to be mentally normal.[8,19,60,63,65,66] The abnormalities are typically nonspecific and include focal or generalized slowing and increases in sharp activity. Both CT and MRI scans, on the other hand, usually appear normal.

More severe parenchymal abnormalities are less common in stage 2, but they do occur in as many as 10 to 20% of patients (see Figure 7–3). When they do, they are accompanied almost always by pleocytosis and, frequently, by meningeal symptoms and cranial or peripheral radiculoneuritis.

MYELITIS

The most frequent severe CNS parenchymal abnormality in stage 2 Lyme disease is myelitis (Figure 7–5),[h] usually an acute or subacute transverse myelitis that develops over hours to days,[i] although the course is sometimes more indolent with increasing deficit over months.[32,64,128] Pleocytosis is almost always (95% of patients) present, and the spinal cord involvement typically begins during an already established meningoradiculitis (85%). Concomitant cerebral involvement is present in about 10%. Both children and adults are affected.

The most common clinical finding is spastic paraparesis with bilateral Babinski signs and loss of superficial reflexes. In acute cases, the paralysis can be flaccid.[23] Spastic quadriparesis has also been reported.[42] There is usually an accompanying sensory loss with a sensory level, most often between T-4 and T-10,[11,19,23,65,70,111] but cervical[31,42] and lumbar[66] sensory levels have been reported occasionally. Autonomic symptoms are also frequent: usually urinary retention or incontinence, fecal incontinence, or impotence. Paraparesis without sensory involvement is common too,[32,42,63,64,78,82,83,128] but isolated sensory myelopathy is rare.[31] Less often, the cord is involved asymmetrically: In two patients there was cervical radiculopathy accompanied by hemihypoesthesia.[31] Milder involvement of the spinal cord is common also: Many patients with stage 2 neurologic disease have isolated Babinski signs, sometimes bilateral, or abnormalities of micturition suggesting spinal cord dysfunction, without other signs of CNS dysfunction (see Figure 7–5).

Radiographic abnormalities in Lyme disease patients with myelitis have been reported infrequently. Myelography is typically normal. MRI has shown cord abnormalities in several patients, including a syrinx in one.[42] Somatosensory-evoked potentials have indicated a demyelinating cord lesion in at least three patients with myelitis,[32,70,128] but have been normal in others.[42]

The prognosis in patients with myelitis is not as good as in patients with peripheral nervous system involvement alone. Residual paraparesis is common, as are disturbances of micturition; at least two patients have been left confined to a wheelchair.[23,66] When improvement does occur, it often takes months.

ENCEPHALITIS

Both children and adults can also suffer more severe cerebral involvement during stage 2 (see Figure 7–5).[j] Encephalitis is almost always accompanied

---

[h]References 11, 12, 19, 23, 31, 32, 42–44, 48, 57, 63–66, 70, 78, 82, 83, 87, 90, 91, 111, 128, 129.
[i]References 11, 19, 23, 31, 42, 43, 48, 65, 70, 86, 87, 111.
[j]References 10–13, 15, 19, 23, 24, 26, 27, 32, 34, 43, 44, 48, 49, 54, 55, 57, 62–64, 66–68, 71, 82, 90, 115, 129.

ABNORMALITY

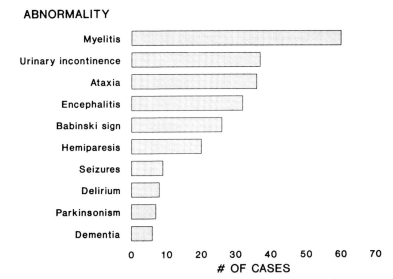

Figure 7–5.   Central nervous system abnormalities during stage 2 Lyme disease.

by pleocytosis (in 95% of cases), and usually by cranial or peripheral radiculo-neuritis (55%), radiculomyelitis (10%), or, rarely, just myelitis (1%). But encephalitis does occur alone (35%) and can be the presenting feature of Lyme disease. When both conditions are present, meningoradiculitis usually precedes encephalitis by days to weeks, but symptoms of both can develop simultaneously, or encephalitis may even appear first. Encephalitis and myelitis usually appear simultaneously when they occur together.

The symptoms typically develop over hours to days (exceptionally, weeks) and include severe somnolence, hallucinatory delirium, disorientation, paranoid psychosis, catatonia, confusion, irritability, and agitation. Coma has been reported in at least five patients,[12,31,49,68,71] and seizures of a variety of types, in at least nine: Partial complex, focal motor, and both primary and secondary generalized convulsive seizures have all been reported.[k]

Focal CNS signs frequently accompany the cerebral symptoms, particularly hemiparesis (see Figure 7–5),[l] which may be either gradual in onset, developing over days to weeks, or sudden, suggesting a vascular cause. Hemianopsia,[31] alexia without agraphia,[10] dysphasia,[10,11] and pseudobulbar palsy have also been reported. In one patient, the locked-in syndrome developed, apparently due to a vascular lesion in the basis pontis.[54] Argyll Robertson pupils have been seen in three others.[45,92,130]

---

[k]References 11, 24, 26, 27, 31, 34, 66, 71, 115.
[l]References 11, 12, 26, 31, 32, 43, 44, 55, 62, 67, 71, 82, 83.

Cerebellar ataxia is even more common than hemiparesis (see Figure 7–5). Ataxia of one limb, hemiataxia, ataxia of stance and gait, and ataxia of all four limbs have all been described.[m] Other reported movement abnormalities include chorea,[65] dystonia,[31] athetosis,[31] and tremor.[74,87]

Parkinson's syndrome can also develop during stage 2.[31,44,48,87,131] The physical findings, which are sometimes asymmetric, include global rigidity, akinesia, hypomimia, tremor, cogwheeling, and postural instability. Symptoms can begin 3 to 12 months after primary infection, develop over weeks to months, and usually improve after antibiotic therapy, sometimes combined temporarily with L-dopa treatment. When Parkinson's syndrome does develop during stage 2 Lyme disease, there is typically an accompanying pleocytosis, sometimes with meningismus, other CNS symptoms or signs, or cranial or peripheral neuritis, all serving to differentiate it from idiopathic Parkinson's disease.

The EEG in patients with severe cerebral symptoms characteristically shows generalized slowing, while focal epileptic abnormalities are present in some patients with seizures. In spite of clinical and EEG evidence for cerebral involvement, the CT and MRI are normal in many patients who have encephalitis clinically. In others, the CT has shown infarct patterns in the cortex and basal ganglia (particularly in patients with hemiparesis)[15,31]; large areas of nonenhancing hypodensity in the white matter with mass effect[71,130]; multifocal areas of white matter abnormality without mass effect, suggesting demyelination (Figure 7–6)[32,130]; low-density contrast-enhancing areas in the cerebral cortex[26]; and, in at least two patients (one with Parkinson's syndrome), hydrocephalus.[31,87] MRI abnormalities have been similar: multiple areas of increased signal in the cerebral and periventricular white matter, and similar areas in the brain stem and the cortical gray matter (Figure 7–7).[23,31] Cerebral angiography in at least two patients with acute encephalitis, and cerebral white matter abnormalities with mass effect on CT, has shown only shift of the anterior cerebral artery without any evidence for vasculitis.[71,130]

Cerebral abnormalities, like those in the spinal cord, resolve more slowly and less completely than those in the peripheral nervous system even after antibiotic treatment. Residual irreversible dementia,[66,130] tetraplegia,[54] cerebral demyelination,[130] and organic psychosis[11,67] have all been reported to follow encephalitis, Parkinson's syndrome does not always resolve completely,[87,131] and hydrocephalus may require shunting despite antibiotic therapy.[87] Persistent hemiparesis[78,82,83] and ataxia[31,83] also occur, as do residual seizures.[26,130]

Myositis

Musculoskeletal symptoms are also common in early disseminated Lyme disease: Over 40% of patients have myalgias, often migratory; 4% experience

---

[m]References 11, 15, 31, 32, 43–45, 65, 67, 71, 74, 82, 83.

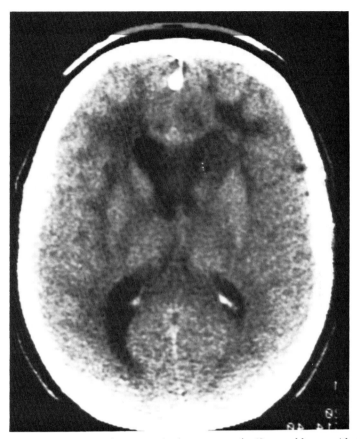

Figure 7–6. Postcontrast cranial computerized tomogram of a 42-year-old man with dementia and partial complex seizures following acute encephalitis during stage 2 Lyme disease. There are extensive areas of low density in the white matter of the frontal lobes compatible with demyelination. (Reproduced with permission from Reik L, Smith L, Khan A, Nelson W. *Neurology* 1985;35:267–269.)

muscle tenderness; and occasional patients have generalized muscle stiffness or severe cramping pain in the muscles of the calves, thighs, or lower and upper back.[3] But muscle weakness is usually absent, and it is not clear how often these symptoms actually indicate muscle inflammation.

In a few patients with stage 2 disease, however, definite myositis has been documented. Duray and Steere referred to a syndrome of severe pain in one or more proximal muscle groups, which they state is "not uncommonly seen in late stage II in Europe."[132] The painful muscles are swollen and tender and show changes of interstitial myositis on biopsy. The myositis can coexist with but is independent of other cardiac muscle or peripheral or central nervous system involvement.

Other European and American authors reported similar histologic

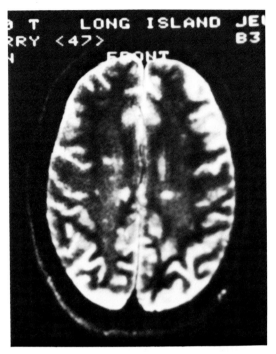

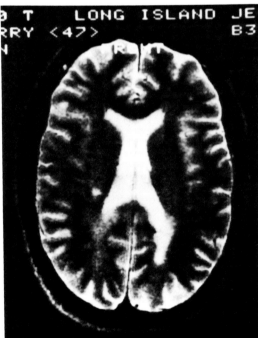

Figure 7–7.   Magnetic resonance images of the brain of a 48-year-old man with severe, acute meningoencephalitis due to Lyme disease. There are multiple areas of increased signal in the white matter on T2-weighted images. (Reproduced with permission from Halperin JJ. *Rheum Dis Clin North Am* 1989;15:635–647.)

findings.[133–140] Symptoms begin 1 week to 6 months after the initial tick bite or EM, and the onset can be either acute or progressive over weeks to months with myalgias, either generalized or localized to one or a few muscle groups, muscle swelling and tenderness, stiffness, and, less often, weakness. Either the arms, the legs, or both can be involved, and the involvement may be asymmetric. Proximal muscles are most often affected, but the distal muscles can be affected as well. Accompanying systemic symptoms are often present and include fever, chills, anorexia, malaise, headache, nausea, and vomiting.

The serum creatine kinase (CK) level may be normal, moderately increased, or increased to several thousand international units. Typical electromyographic abnormalities are polyphasic, short-duration, low-amplitude action potentials; positive sharp waves; and fibrillation potentials. In patients with concomitant peripheral nerve involvement, long-duration, high-amplitude potentials; slowing of NCV; and prolonged distal latencies may also be present. In two patients, gallium 67 imaging showed intense uptake of radiotracer in the affected muscles.[133,135]

Antibiotic treatment is curative, with resolution of pain in weeks and weakness within a month or two.

Stage 2 Neuroborreliosis in Children

B. burgdorferi can cross the placenta during pregnancy and cause both fetal demise and fatal congenital infection in the newborn, with organisms present in the meninges, subarachnoid space, and brain at necropsy.[141,142] But no consistent pattern of congenital malformation has been linked to intrauterine infection, and no progressive neurologic illness after birth has been described following infection of the mother during pregnancy.[143]

Acquired Lyme disease, on the other hand, is quite common during childhood. The incidence of Lyme disease in children aged 5 to 9 is greater than that in adults aged 20 to 24 years[144]; in Westchester County, New York, 40% of reported cases are in children age 19 or younger.[145] The general features of the illness do not differ substantially from those in adults, although fever may be more likely in childhood cases, joint complaints may be more common, antecedent tick bites may be recalled more often, and EM may be less frequent.[145] Boys are affected more often than girls.

Early (stage 2) neurologic involvement occurs in about 15% of childhood cases,[145] but the clinical course is often milder and shorter than in adults.[19,63,82] Aseptic meningitis, with severe headache and slight neck stiffness, and facial palsy (usually with pleocytosis) are the most common neurologic abnormalities.[19,37,40,55,63,82,98] The CSF abnormalities are no different than those in adults. Typical painful radiculitis is rare in children with neuroborelliosis, however: None of the 66 pediatric cases from Germany investigated by Christen et al. had Bannwarth's syndrome.[98]

Yet more severe neurologic abnormalities do occur during early Lyme disease in children. Bannwarth's syndrome has been recorded in a number of patients,[16,63,74] and parenchymal CNS involvement can develop. Mild cerebral symptoms, chorea, ataxia, severe encephalitis, seizures, coma, hemiparesis, and transverse myelitis have all been reported,[19,26,55,65,71,74,98] although less often than in adults. While nervous system involvement in Lyme disease in children is generally more benign than in adults, it appears, therefore, that children can suffer the whole range of neurologic abnormalities described in older patients.

European Versus North American Early Lyme Disease

Early reports of Lyme disease from North America emphasized a number of differences from European EM and related disorders. Nervous system involvement was thought to be less common and to be preceded more often by EM in North America, and Lyme arthritis was believed not to occur in Europe.[2,60,65]

As neuroborreliosis does develop without antecedent EM in the United States,[66] and Lyme arthritis does occur in Europe,[5,6,146] these reported differences probably resulted, at least in part, from ascertainment bias and differences in treatment between the two continents.[147] Early North American reports described prospective studies of patients with either EM or arthritis and therefore overestimated the frequency of both. Early European reports concentrated on Bannwarth's syndrome, overestimating its frequency and underestimating that of EM. In addition, the European practice of treating EM with oral antibiotics, common there since the 1940s but not routine in the United States until the 1980s, may have lowered the frequency of arthritis among European patients compared to that of neurologic involvement, since such early treatment can prevent later arthritis but may not eliminate all organisms from the nervous system.[147]

However, arthritis is probably still more common among North American than European patients, and some other general clinical differences that remain could relate to variations among strains of *B. burgdorferi* from the two continents. Åsbrink et al. showed in a careful prospective study that multiple secondary skin lesions, severe systemic symptoms, and laboratory abnormalities are less common in Swedish patients with EM than in those from North America, while a prolonged course (> 6 months) of EM is more common.[148] Moreover, lymphocytoma appears to be almost uniquely European.[6,146]

Other unreconciled differences between the patterns of early neurologic abnormalities on the two continents may also relate to strain variation. The initial report of nervous system involvement in North American Lyme disease emphasized the frequency of mild cerebral symptoms, which had not been reported in European patients.[65] A subsequent American report did find these symptoms to be less frequent,[60] and the frequency of severe CNS involvement does not differ between the two; but, it is still not clear whether the brain is involved more often in North American patients or whether milder cerebral symptoms have not been sought as carefully in European patients.

Similarly, meningeal symptoms seem to be more frequent and more profound in North American patients with pleocytosis among whom headache is intense, long lasting, and nearly universal and meningismus frequent.[60,65,66] Early European reports, however, described the meningitis of Bannwarth's syndrome as often asymptomatic.[8,94] Although more recent reports from Europe indicate a higher frequency of symptomatic meningitis,[n] a substantial discrepancy remains.

Finally, there appear to be differences in the relationship between the site of the initiating tick bite or EM and subsequent radicular pain and motor weakness in meningopolyneuritis. Many, but not all, European reports of Bannwarth's syndrome indicate that the radicular pain usually begins in and is more severe in the same dermatomal segment as the bite and ensuing EM[13,25,56,63,85,94] as is the later motor weakness.[34,83,89] Reports from North America have not confirmed this relationship.

References

1. Allal J, Thomas Ph, Mazzonelli H. Borrelia isolated from cerebrospinal fluid in a French case of Lyme disease. *Ann Rheum Dis* 1986;45:789–790.
2. Steere AC, Malawista SE, Hardin JA, Ruddy S, Askenase PW, Andiman WA. Erythema chronicum migrans and Lyme arthritis: The enlarging clinical spectrum. *Ann Intern Med* 1977;86:685–698.
3. Steere AC, Bartenhagen NH, Craft JE, et al. The early clinical manifestations of Lyme disease. *Ann Intern Med* 1983;99:76–82.
4. Steere AC, Malawista SE, Bartenhagen NH, et al. The clinical spectrum and treatment of Lyme disease. *Yale J Biol Med* 1984;57:453–461.
5. Åsbrink E, Olsson I, Hovmark A. Erythema chronicum migrans Afzelius in Sweden: A study of 231 patients. *Zentralbl Bakteriol Mikrobiol Hyg [A]* 1986;263:229–236.
6. Weber K, Neubert U. Clinical features of early erythema migrans disease and related disorders. *Zentralbl Bakteriol Mikrobiol Hyg [A]* 1986;263:209–228.
7. Kuiper H, de Jongh B, Ramselaar T, Spanjaard L. Evidence of asymptomatic nervous system involvement in localized erythema migrans. Presented at the Fourth International Conference on Lyme Borreliosis; June 18–21, 1990; Stockholm, Sweden.
8. Ackermann R, Horstrup P, Schmidt R. Tick-borne meningopolyneuritis (Garin-Bujadoux-Bannwarth). *Yale J Biol Med* 1984;57:485–490.
9. Åsbrink E, Olsson I, Hovmark A, Carlsson B. Tick-borne spirochetes as a cause of facial palsy. *Clin Otolaryngol* 1985;10:279–284.
10. Bataillard M, Bernard C, Cardey A, Cotte Rittaud M, Hanhart R. Atteinte prédominante du système nerveux central au cours d'une forme secondaire de borreliose. *Rev Neurol (Paris)* 1988;10:610–611.
11. Bateman DE, Lawton NF, White JE, Greenwood RJ, Wright DJM. The neurological complications of *Borrelia burgdorferi* in the New Forest area of Hampshire. *J Neurol Neurosurg Psychiatry* 1988;51:699–703.
12. Baumhackl U, Kristoferitsch W, Sluga E, Stanek G. Neurological manifestations of *Borrelia burgdorferi*–infections: The enlarging clinical spectrum. *Zentralbl Bakteriol Mikrobiol Hyg [A]* 1986;263:334–336.

---

[n]References 12, 19, 20, 34, 40, 44, 55, 63, 81, 82, 87.

13. Boudin G, Vernant J-C, Lanoé et Vojir Y. Les paralysies par morsure de tiques: arbovirose ou origine toxinique? *Ann Med Interne (Paris)* 1974;125:55–60.
14. Bourdel A, Viader F, Dupuy B, et al. Maladie de Lyme révélée par une polyradiculonévrite sans hypercytose du liquide céphalorachidien. *Presse Med* 1988;17:1214–1215.
15. Bourke SJ, Baird AG, Bone FJ, Baird DR, Stevenson RD. Lyme disease with acute purulent meningitis. *Br Med J* 1988;297:460.
16. Caflisch U, Tönz O, Schaad UB, Aeschlimann A, Burgdorfer W. Die Zecken-Meningo-radikulitis—eine Spirochätose. *Schweiz Med Wochenschr* 1984;114:630–634.
17. Camponovo F, Meier C. Neuropathy of vasculitic origin in a case of Garin-Boujadoux-Bannwarth syndrome with positive borrelia antibody response. *J Neurol* 1986;233:69–72.
18. Clark JR, Carlson RD, Sasaki CT, Pachner AR, Steere AC. Facial paralysis in Lyme disease. *Laryngoscope* 1985;95:1341–1345.
19. Christen H-J, Hanefeld F. Neurologic complications of erythema-migrans-disease in childhood—clinical aspects. *Zentralbl Bakteriol Mikrobiol Hyg [A]* 1986;263:337–342.
20. Christen H-J, Bartlau N, Hanefeld F, Thomssen R. Lyme-Borreliose—häufigste Ursache der akuten peripheren Fazialisparese im Kindesalter. *Monatsschr Kinderheilkd* 1989;137:151–157.
21. Daffner KR, Saver JL, Biber MP. Lyme polyradiculoneuropathy presenting as increasing abdominal girth. *Neurology* 1990;40:373–375.
22. Dekonenko EJ, Steere AC, Berardi VP, Kravchuk LN. Lyme borreliosis in the Soviet Union: A cooperative US-USSR report. *J Infect Dis* 1988;158:748–753.
23. Di Bella P, Logullo F, Dionisi L, Testa I, Angeleri F. Meningoencephalomyeloradiculo-neuritis in one case of *Borrelia burgdorferi* infection (Lyme disease). *Ital J Neurol Sci* 1989;10:457–461.
24. Diringer MN, Halperin JJ, Dattwyler RJ. Lyme meningoencephalitis: Report of a severe penicillin-resistant case. *Arthritis Rheum* 1987;30:705–708.
25. Dupuis M, Mertens C, Gonsette RE, Nuytten W, Bouffioux J, Dobbelaere F. Méningo-radiculite par spirochète (*Borrelia burgdorferi*) après piqûre d'arthropodes. *Rev Neurol (Paris)* 1985;141:780–785.
26. Feder HM, Zalneraitis EL, Reik L. Lyme disease: Acute focal meningoencephalitis in a child. *Pediatrics* 1988;82:931–934.
27. Ferroir JP, Reignier A, Nicolle MH, Guillard A. Méningo-radiculo-névraxite de la maladie de Lyme: un cas avec troubles mentaux majeurs et régressifs. *Presse Med* 1988;17:697.
28. Garin C, Bujadoux C. Paralysie par les Tiques. *J Med Lyon* 1922;71:765–767.
29. Graf M, Kristoferitsch W, Baumhackl U, Zeitlhofer J. Electrophysiologic findings in men-ingopolyneuritis of Garin-Bujadoux-Bannwarth. *Zentralbl Bakteriol Mikrobiol Hyg [A]* 1986;263:324–327.
30. Hanner P, Rosenhall U, Edström S, Kaijser B. Hearing impairment in patients with antibody production against *Borrelia burgdorferi* antigen. *Lancet* 1989;1:13–15.
31. Hänny PE, Häuselmann HJ. Die Lyme-Krankheit aus der Sicht des Neurologen. *Schweiz Med Wochenschr* 1987;117:901–915.
32. Hansen K, Rechnitzer C, Pedersen NS, Arpi M, Jessen O. *Borrelia* meningitis in Denmark. *Zentralbl Bakteriol Mikrobiol Hyg [A]* 1986;263:348–350.
33. Hindfelt B, Jeppsson PG, Nillson B, Olsson J-E, Ryberg B, Sörnäs R. Clinical and cerebro-spinal fluid findings in lymphocytic meningoradiculitis (Bannwarth's syndrome). *Acta Neurol Scand* 1982;66:444–453.
34. Hirsch E, Sellal F, Christmann D, et al. Les méningoradiculites après morsure de tique: étude de 31 cas. *Rev Neurol (Paris)* 1987;143:182–188.
35. Hofstad H, Nyland H. Bannwarth's syndrome and its relation to Lyme disease. *Acta Neurol Scan* 1984;70:381.
36. Hugon J, Vallat JM, Outrequin G, Dumas M, Desproges-Gotteron R. Méningoradiculo-neuropathies après piqures de tiques; étude électrophysiologique de 7 observations. *Lyon Med* 1984;15:305–306.
37. Huppertz H-I, Sticht-Groh V. Meningitis due to *Borrelia burgdorferi* in the initial stage of Lyme disease. *Eur J Pediatr* 1989;148:428–430.
38. Jesel M, Isch-Treussard C, Warter JM, Coquillat G, Roos M. Méningoradiculites et poly-radiculonévrites: corrélations cliniques et E.M.G. *Rev Electroencephalogr Neurophysiol Clin* 1975;5:406–410.
39. Jonsson L, Stiernstedt G, Thomander L. Tick-borne *Borrelia* infection in patients with Bell's palsy. *Arch Otolaryngol Head Neck Surg* 1987;113:303–306.
40. Jörbeck HJA, Gustafsson PM, Lind HCF, Stiernstedt GT. Tick-borne *Borrelia*-meningitis in

children: An outbreak in the Kalmar area during the summer of 1984. *Acta Paediatr Scand* 1987;76:228–233.
41. Klöter I, Adam T, Schabet M, Wiethölter H, Peiffer J. Borrelia-induced meningoradiculitis—two different forms of the disease. *Eur Neurol* 1986;25:262–268.
42. Kohler J. Lyme borreliosis: A case of transverse myelitis with syrinx cavity. *Neurology* 1989;39:1553–1554.
43. Kohlhepp W, Mertens H-G, Oschmann P. Acute and chronic illness after tick-bite *Borrelia burgdorferi*–infections: Results of treatment. *Zentralbl Bakteriol Mikrobiol Hyg [A]* 1986; 263:365–371.
44. Kohlhepp W, Mertens HG, Oschmann P, Rohrback E. Akute und chronische Erkrankungen bei zeckenvermittelter Borreliose. *Nervenarzt* 1987;58:557–563.
45. Koudstaal PJ, Vermeulen M, Wokke JHJ. Argyll Robertson pupils in lymphocytic meningoradiculitis (Bannwarth's syndrome). *J Neurol Neurosurg Psychiatry* 1987;50:363–365.
46. Krejcova H, Bojar M, Jerabek J, Tomas J, Jirous J. Otoneurological symtomatology in Lyme disease. *Adv Otorhinolaryngol* 1988;42:210–212.
47. Kristoferitsch W, Baumhackl U, Sluga E, Stanek G, Zeiler K. High-dose penicillin therapy in meningopolyneuritis Garin-Bujadoux-Bannwarth: Clinical and cerebrospinal fluid data. *Zentralbl Bakteriol Mikrobiol Hyg [A]* 1986;263:357–364.
48. Krüger H, Reuss K, Pulz M, et al. Meningoradiculitis and encephalomyelitis due to *Borrelia burgdorferi*: A follow-up study of 72 patients over 27 years. *J Neurol* 1989;236:322–328.
49. Louis FJ, Schill H, Le Bris H, et al. Deux formes neurologiques graves de maladie de Lyme. *Presse Med* 1987;16:32–33.
50. Lubeau M, Vallat JM, Hugon J, Dumas M, Desproges-Gotteron R. Tick bite meningoradiculitis: Ten cases. *Zentralbl Bakteriol Mikrobiol Hyg [A]* 1986;263:321–323.
51. Markby DP. Lyme disease facial palsy: Differentiation from Bell's palsy. *Br Med J* 1989;299:605–606.
52. Meier C, Grehl H. Vaskulitische Neuropathie bei Garin-Bujadoux-Bannwarth-Syndrom: ein Beitrag zum Verständnis der Pathologie und Pathogenese neurologischer Komplikationen bei Lyme-Borreliose. *Dtsch Med Wochenschr* 1988;113:135–138.
53. Melet M, Gerard A, Voiriot P, et al. Méningoradiculonévrite mortelle au cours d'une maladie de Lyme. *Presse Med* 1986;15:2075.
54. Merlo A, Weder B, Ketz E, Matter L. Locked-in state in *Borrelia burgdorferi* meningitis. *J Neurol* 1989;236:305–306.
55. Lyme borreliosis in children: A controlled study based on ELISA values. *Eur J Pediatr* 1989;148:527–530.
56. Morin B, Dordain G, Tournilhac M, Rey M. Méningoradiculites après piqûre de tique. *Presse Med* 1976;5:1965–1968.
57. Muhlemann MF, Wright DJM. Emerging pattern of Lyme disease in the United Kingdom and Irish Republic. *Lancet* 1987;1:260–262.
58. Olsson I, Engervall K, Åsbrink E, Carlsson-Nordlander B, Hovmark A. Tick-borne borreliosis and facial palsy. *Acta Otolaryngol (Stockh)* 1988;105:100–107.
59. Pachner AR, Steere AC. Neurologic findings of Lyme disease. *Yale J Biol Med* 1984;57:481–483.
60. Pachner AR, Steere AC. The triad of neurologic manifestations of Lyme disease: Meningitis, cranial neuritis and radiculoneuritis. *Neurology* 1985;35:47–53.
61. Pal GS, Baker JT, Wright DJM. Penicillin-resistant *Borrelia* encephalitis responding to cefotaxime. *Lancet* 1988;1:50–51.
62. Pfister HW, Einhäupl K, Preac-Mursic B, Wilske B, Schierz G. The spirochetal etiology of lymphocytic meningoradiculitis of Bannwarth (Bannwarth's syndrome). *J Neurol* 1984; 231:141–144.
63. Pfister HW, Einhäupl KM, Wilske B, Preac-Mursic V. Bannwarth's syndrome and the enlarged neurological spectrum of arthropod-borne borreliosis. *Zentralbl Bakteriol Mikrobiol Hyg [A]* 1986;263:343–347.
64. Poullot B, Marmonier A, Haas C, Dournon E. La méningoradiculite à tique et autres aspects neurologiques de la maladie de Lyme. *Rev Med Interne* 1987;8:350–356.
65. Reik L, Steere AC, Bartenhagen NH, Shope RE, Malawista SE. Neurologic abnormalities of Lyme disease. *Medicine (Baltimore)* 1979;58:281–294.
66. Reik L, Burgdorfer W, Donaldson JO. Neurologic abnormalities in Lyme disease without erythema chronicum migrans. *Am J Med* 1986;81:73–78.
67. Riedmann G, Barolin GS. Neuroborreliose. *Wien Med Wochenschr* 1988;138:613–616.
68. Rohmer F, Collard M, Jesel M, Warter JM, Coquillat G, Class JJ. Les méningoradiculites:

données cliniques, électromyographiques et étiologiques à propos de 36 observations: limites nosologiques. *Rev Neurol* 1974;130:415–431.

69. Rosenhall U, Hanner P, Kaijser B. Borrelia infection and vertigo. *Acta Otolaryngol (Stockh)* 1988;106:111–116.

70. Rousseau JJ, Lust C, Zangerle PF, Bigaignon G. Acute transverse myelitis as presenting neurological feature of Lyme disease. *Lancet* 1986;2:1222–1223.

71. Rousselle C, Floret D, Cochat P, Reignier F, Wright C. Encéphalite aiguë à *Borrelia burgdorferi* (maladie de Lyme) chez un enfant algérien. *Pediatrie* 1989;44:265–269.

72. Rybert B. Bannwarth's syndrome (lymphocytic meningoradiculitis) in Sweden. *Yale J Biol Med* 1984;57:499–503.

73. Schechter SL. Lyme disease associated with optic neuropathy. *Am J Med* 1986;81:143–145.

74. Schmedding E, Verboven M, Lauwers S, Ebinger G, Rom N, Loeb H. Lymphocytic meningoradiculitis (Garin-Bujadoux-Bannwarth): From syndrome to disease? *Eur J Pediatr* 1986;144:497–502.

75. Schmutzhard E, Stanek G, Pohl P. Polyneuritis cranialis associated with *Borrelia burgdorferi*. *J Neurol Neurosurg Psychiatry* 1985;48:1182–1184.

76. Schmutzhard E, Pohl P, Stanek G. Involvement of *Borrelia burgdorferi* in cranial nerve affection. *Zentralbl Bakteriol Mikrobiol Hyg [A]* 1986;263:328–333.

77. Sindic CJM, Depre A, Bigaignon G, Goubau PF, Hella P, Laterre C. Lymphocytic meningoradiculitis and encephalomyelitis due to *Borrelia burgdorferi*: A clinical and serological study of 18 cases. *J Neurol Neurosurg Psychiatry* 1987;50:1565–1571.

78. Sköldenberg B, Stiernstedt G, Gårde A, Kolmodin G, Carlström A, Nord CE. Chronic meningitis caused by a penicillin-sensitive microorganism? *Lancet* 1983;2:75–78.

79. Steere AC, Pachner AR, Malawista SE. Neurologic abnormalities of Lyme disease: Successful treatment with high-dose intravenous penicillin. *Ann Intern Med* 1983;99:767–772.

80. Sterman AB, Nelson S, Barclar P. Demyelinating neuropathy accompanying Lyme disease. *Neurology* 1982;32:1302–1305.

81. Stiernstedt G. Tick-borne borrelia infection in Sweden. *Scand J Infect Dis Suppl* 1985;45:1–70.

82. Stiernstedt GT, Sköldenberg BR, Gårde A, et al. Clinical manifestations of *Borrelia* infections of the nervous system. *Zentralbl Bakteriol Bakteriol Hyg [A]* 1986;263:289–296.

83. Stiernstedt G, Gustafsson R, Karlsson M, Svenungsson B, Sköldenberg B. Clinical manifestations and diagnosis of neuroborreliosis. *Ann NY Acad Sci* 1988;539:46–55.

84. Uldry PA, Steck AJ, Regli F. Manifestations neurologiques des infections à *Borrelia burgdorferi*. *Schweiz Med Wochenschr* 1986;116:135–142.

85. Vallat JM, Hugon J, Lubeau M, Leboutet MJ, Dumas M, Desproges-Gotteron R. Tick-bite meningoradiculoneuritis: Clinical, electrophysiologic, and histologic findings in 10 cases. *Neurology* 1987;37:749–753.

86. Vandvik B, Sköldenberg B, Stiernstedt G. Tick-borne spirochaetal meningitis, meningoradiculitis and meningoencephalitis: A report on 15 cases identified by demonstration of intrathecal spirochaete-specific IgG antibody responses. *Acta Neurol Scand* 1984;70:379–380.

87. Viader R, Poncelet AM, Chapon F, et al. Les formes neurologiques de la maladie de Lyme: 12 cas. *Rev Neurol* 1989;145:362–368.

88. Vickerfors T, Rudbäck N. Borrelia meningoradiculitis with severe pains. *Scand J Infect Dis* 1987;19:701–702.

89. Vieyres C, Allal J, Coisne D, Thomas P, Neau JP, Breux JP. Aspects européens de la maladie de Lyme: huit cas. *Presse Med* 1987;16:59–62.

90. Wenig C. Chronische lymphozytäre Meningitis mit polytoper Beteilung des Nervensystems (nach Zeckenbiss?). *Psychiatr Neurol Med Psychol (Leipz)* 1975;27:592–600.

91. Wokke JHJ, Burgdorfer W. Bannwarth's syndrome in the Netherlands. *Zentralbl Bakteriol Mikrobiol Hyg [A]* 1986;263:351.

92. Wokke JHJ, van Doorn PA, Brand A, Schreuder GMT, Vermeulen M. Association of HLA-DR2 antigen with serum IgG antibodies against *Borrelia burgdorferi* in Bannwarth's syndrome. *J Neurol* 1988;235:415–417.

93. Wulff CH, Hansen K, Strange P, Trojabord W. Multiple mononeuritis and radiculitis with erythema, pain, elevated CSF protein and pleocytosis (Bannwarth's syndrome). *J Neurol Neurosurg Psychiatry* 1983;46:485–490.

94. Hörstrup P, Ackermann R. Durch Zecken übertragene Meningopolyneuritis (Garin-Bujadoux-Bannwarth). *Fortschr Neurol Psychiatr* 1973;41:583–606.

95. Meyer-Rienecker HJ, Hitzschke B. Lymphocytic meningoradiculitis. In: Vinken PJ, Bruyn GW, eds. *Handbook of Clinical Neurology* New York: Elsevier; 1978;34:571–586.

96. Herskowitz S, Berger A, Swerdlow ML. Guillain-Barré syndrome associated with Lyme borreliosis. *Neurology* 1990;40(suppl 1):342.
97. Bourdel A, Viader F, Dupuy B, et al. Maladie de Lyme révélée par une polyradiculonévrite sans hypercytose du liquide céphalorachidien. *Presse Med* 1988;17:1214–1215.
98. Christen H-J, Eiffert H, Lotter H, Scriba M, Hanefeld F. Facial palsy and aseptic meningitis caused by *Borrelia burgdorferi*: Report on an ongoing prospective study in childhood. Presented at the Fourth International Conference on Lyme Borreliosis; June 18–21, 1990; Stockholm, Sweden.
99. Bouma PAD, Carpay HA. Antibodies to *Borrelia burgdorferi* in Guillain-Barré syndrome. *Lancet* 1989;2:739.
100. Mancardi GL, Del Sette M, Primavera A, Farinelli M, Fumarola D. A prospective study of acute idiopathic neuropathy II antecedent events. *J Neurol Neurosurg Psychiatry* 1989; 52:424–425.
101. Mancardi GL, Del Sette M, Primavera A, Farinelli M, Fumarola D. *Borrelia burgdorferi* infection and Guillain-Barré syndrome. *Lancet* 1989;2:985–986.
102. Baumhackl U, Kristoferitsch W, Pilz P, et al. Intrathecally synthesized antibodies to *Borrelia burgdorferi* in facial palsy: A multicenter study. Presented at the Fourth International Conference on Lyme Borreliosis; June 18–21, 1990; Stockholm, Sweden.
103. Engervall K, Hederstedt B, Hovmark A, et al. Borreliosis as a cause of peripheral facial palsy in Sweden: A multicenter study. Presented at the Fourth International Conference on Lyme Borreliosis; June 18–21, 1990; Stockholm, Sweden.
104. Halperin JJ, Golightly M. Lyme borreliosis in Bell's palsy. *Neurology* 1990;40(suppl 1):342.
105. Roberg M, Forsberg P, Frydén A, et al. Serological long-term follow up of untreated patients with facial palsy using two different *Borrelia burgdorferi* antigens. Presented at the Fourth International Conference on Lyme Borreliosis; June 18–21, 1990; Stockholm, Sweden.
106. Lind O, Ekstrand T. Borrelia serology in patients with facial palsy in a region with a low rate of ticks. Presented at the Fourth International Conference on Lyme Borreliosis; June 18–21, 1990; Stockholm, Sweden.
107. Kuiper H, Devriese P, de Jongh B. Lyme borreliosis and Bell's palsy: A prospective study in 69 patients in the Netherlands. Presented at the Fourth International Conference on Lyme Borreliosis; June 18–21, 1990; Stockholm, Sweden.
108. Raucher HS, Kaufman DM, Goldfarb J, Jacobson RI, Roseman B, Wolff RR. Pseudotumor cerebri and Lyme disease: A new association. *J Pediatr* 1985;107:931–933.
109. Wu G, Lincoff H, Ellsworth RM, Haik BG. Optic disc edema and Lyme disease. *Ann Ophthalmol* 1986;18:252–255.
110. Jacobson DM, Frens DB. Psuedotumor cerebri syndrome associated with Lyme disease. *Am J Ophthalmol* 1989;107:81–82.
111. Farris BK, Webb RM. Lyme disease and optic neuritis. *J Clin Neuro Ophthalmol* 1988;8:73–78.
112. Gustafson R, Svenungsson B. Optic neuropathy in *Borrelia* infection. *J Infect* 1988;17:187–188.
113. Schönherr U, Wilk CM, Lang G, Naumann GOH. Intraocular manifestations of Lyme borreliosis. Presented at the Fourth International Conference on Lyme Borreliosis; June 18–21, 1990; Stockholm, Sweden.
114. Schroeter V, Belz GG, Blenk H. Paralysis of recurrent laryngeal nerve in Lyme disease. *Lancet* 1988;2:1245.
115. Pal GS, Baker JT, Humphrey PRD. Lyme disease presenting as recurrent acute meningitis. *Br Med J* 1987;295:367.
116. Razavi-Encha F, Fleury-Feith J, Gherardi R, Bernaudin J-F. Cytologic features of cerebrospinal fluid in Lyme disease. *Acta Cytol (Baltimore)* 1987;31:439–440.
117. Pohl P, Schmutzhard E, Stanek G. Cerebrospinal fluid findings in neurological manifestations of Lyme disease. *Zentralbl Bakteriol Mikrobiol Hyg [A]* 1986;263:314–320.
118. Krüger H, Englert D, Pflughaupt K-W. Demonstration of oligoclonal immunoglobulin G in Guillain-Barré syndrome and lymphocytic meningoradiculitis by isoelectric focusing. *J Neurol* 1981;226:15–24.
119. Maida E, Kristoferitsch W, Spiel G. Liquorveränderungen bei Meningoradiculitis Garin-Bujadoux-Bannwarth. *Nervenarzt* 1986;57:149–152.
120. Szyfelbein WM, Ross JS. Lyme disease meningopolyneuritis simulating malignant lymphoma. *Mod Pathol* 1988;1:464–468.
121. Kristoferitsch W, Steck AJ, Murray N, Stanek G, Lanschützer H. Oligoclonal antibodies in CSF of patients with meningopolyneuritis Garin-Bujadoux-Bannwarth: Ig class, light chain type and specificity. *Zentralbl Bakteriol Mikrobiol Hyg [A]* 1986;263:307–313.
122. Kristoferitsch W, Landschützer H. Oligoklonales Immunglobulin M im Liquor cerbro-

spinalis von Patienten mit Meningopolyneuritis Garin-Bujadoux-Bannwarth. *Wien Klin Wochenschr* 1986;12:386–387.

123. Hansen K, Cruz M, Link H. Oligoclonal *Borrelia burgdorferi*–specific IgG antibodies in cerebrospinal fluid in Lyme neuroborreliosis. *J Infect Dis* 1990;161:1194–1202.

124. Henriksson A, Link J, Cruz M, Stiernstedt G. Immunoglobulin abnormalities in cerebrospinal fluid and blood over the course of lymphocytic meningoradiculitis (Bannwarth's syndrome). *Ann Neurol* 1986;20:337–345.

125. Felgenhauer K. Differentiation of the humoral immune response in inflammatory diseases of the central nervous system. *J Neurol* 1982;228:223–237.

126. Boeer A, Schipper HI, Prange HW. Local IgM production in meningoradiculitis Bannwarth and neurosyphilis. *J Neuroimmunol* 1988;20:315–316.

127. Murray N, Kristoferitsch W, Stanek G, Steck AJ. Specificity of CSF antibodies against components of *Borrelia burgdorferi* in patients with meningopolyneuritis Garin-Bujadoux-Bannwarth. *J Neurol* 1986;233:224–227.

128. Benoit P, Dournon E, Masingue M, Destee A, Warot P. Méningonévraxite borrélienne: un cas. *Presse Med* 1987;16:1733–1736.

129. Schmidt R, Kabatzki J, Hartung S, Ackermann R. Erythema-migrans-Borreliose in der Bundesrepublik Deutschland. *Dtsch Med Wochenschr* 1985;110:1803–1807.

130. Reik L, Smith L, Khan A, Nelson W. Demyelinating encephalopathy in Lyme disease. *Neurology* 1985;35:267–269.

131. Kohlhepp W, Kuhn W, Krüger H. Extrapyramidal features in central Lyme borreliosis. *Eur Neurol* 1989;29:150–155.

132. Duray PH, Steere AC. Clinical pathologic correlations of Lyme disease by stage. *Ann NY Acad Sci* 1988;539:65–79.

133. Atlas E, Novak SN, Duray PH, Steere AC. Lyme myositis: Muscle invasion by *Borrelia burgdorferi*. *Ann Intern Med* 1988;109:245–246.

134. Del Sette M, Caponnetto C, Fumarola D, Mancardi GL. Unusual neurological manifestations of Lyme disease: A case report. *Ital J Neurol Sci* 1989;10:455–456.

135. Kengen RAM, Linde MV, Sprenger HG, Piers DA. Scintigraphic evaluation of Lyme disease: Gallium-67 imaging of Lyme myositis. *Clin Nucl Med* 1989;14:728–729.

136. Kirsch M, Ruben FL, Steere AC, Duray PH, Norden CW, Winkelstein A. Fatal adult respiratory distress syndrome in a patient with Lyme disease. *JAMA* 1988;259:2737–2739.

137. Reimers CD, Pongratz DE, Neubert U, et al. Myositis caused by *Borrelia burgdorferi*: Report of four cases. *J Neurol Sci* 1989;91:215–226.

138. Reimers CD, de Koning J, Pilz A, et al. Myositis associated with *Borrelia burgdorferi*–infection. Presented at the Fourth International Conference on Lyme Borreliosis; June 18–21, 1990; Stockholm, Sweden.

139. Schmutzhard E, Willeit J, Gerstenbrand F. Meningopolyneuritis Bannwarth with focal nodular myositis: A new aspect in Lyme borreliosis. *Klin Wochenschr* 1986;64:1204–1208.

140. Schoenen J, Sianard-Gainko, Carpentier M, Reznik M. Myositis during *Borrelia burgdorferi* infection (Lyme disease). *J Neurol Neurosurg Psychiatry* 1989;52:1002–1005.

141. MacDonald AB, Benach JL, Burgdorfer W. Stillbirth following maternal Lyme disease. *NY State J Med* 1987;87:615–616.

142. Weber K, Bratzke H-J, Neubert U, Wilske B, Duray PH. *Borrelia burgdorferi* in a newborn despite oral penicillin for Lyme borreliosis during pregnancy. *Pediatr Infect Dis J* 1988;7:286–289.

143. Zalneraitis EL, Gerber MA. Prevalence of clinically significant neurologic disorders attributable to congenital Lyme disease. Presented at the Fourth International Conference on Lyme Disease; June 18–21, 1990; Stockholm, Sweden.

144. Belani K, Regelmann WE. Lyme disease in children. *Rheum Dis Clin North Am* 1989;15:679–690.

145. Williams CL, Strobino B, Lee A, et al. Lyme disease in childhood: Clinical and epidemiologic features of ninety cases. *Pediatr Infect Dis J* 1990;9:10–14.

146. Huaux JP, Bignaignon G, Stadtsbaeder S, Zangerle PF, de Deuxchaisnes CN. Pattern of Lyme arthritis in Europe: Report of 14 cases. *Ann Rheum Dis* 1988;47:164–165.

147. Dattwyler RJ, Volkman DJ, Luft BJ, Halperin JJ. Lyme disease in Europe and North America. *Lancet* 1987;1:681.

148. Åsbrink E, Olsson I. Clinical manifestations of erythema chronicum migrans Afzelius in 161 patients: A comparison with Lyme disease. *Acta Derm Venereol (Stockh)* 1985;65:43–52.

149. Åsbrink E, Hovmark A. Early and late cutaneous manifestations in *Ixodes*-borne borreliosis (erythema migrans borreliosis, Lyme borreliosis). *Ann NY Acad Sci* 1988;539:4–15.

8

Neurologic Abnormalities in Late Lyme Disease

A variety of neurologic abnormalities, both central and peripheral, can develop during late Lyme disease, often after an asymptomatic interval. Accumulating evidence now suggests that these abnormalities result from the persistence of live spirochetes in the nervous system. Once *Borrelia burgdorferi* penetrates the nervous system, it can remain there for months to years, either latent or causing disease. The spirochete has been cultured from the normal, uninflamed CSF of an asymptomatic, seropositive patient[1]; cultured from the CSF of a patient with meningopolyneuritis 9 months after a preceding erythema migrans (EM)[2]; and demonstrated by silver staining of the CSF sediment of another patient 15 months after the onset of chronic meningopolyneuritis.[3]

Central Nervous System Abnormalities

Progressive Borrelia Encephalomyelitis

The best defined late nervous system abnormality in Lyme disease is progressive borrelia encephalomyelitis, a syndrome most common in Europe where it has now been reported from a number of countries.[a]

---

[a] Unless otherwise noted, the information presented in this section is derived from data compiled from previous reports[3–38] which contain 140 cases of progressive borrelia encephalomyelitis reported from Belgium, Germany, France, Italy, the Netherlands, Norway, Sweden, Switzerland, and the United States.

The average age at onset is 45 years (range, 7 to 79 years), and the male-to-female ratio among those affected is 1.5:1. While it is usually not possible to determine the interval between initial infection and the beginning of neurologic symptoms, in 9% of cases a tick bite (7%) or other insect "sting" (2%) preceded the onset by 10 days to 19 months (median, 7 months).[b] Seven cases followed EM by 4 months to 6 years (median, 15 months),[8,11,13,25,30,35,38] and, one other, acrodermatitis chronica atrophicans (ACA) by 1 year.[38] In 14% of cases, either a stage 2 meningopolyneuritis (13%) or meningitis alone (1%) was present 3 months to 7 years before onset (median, 12 months).[c] Other less specific antecedent illnesses have included rash[10]; uveitis accompanied by systemic symptoms and pleocytosis[38]; fever, myalgia, and pharyngitis[18]; and a flu-like illness and arthritis[30] days to 5 years before the first symptoms of encephalomyelitis.

Symptoms have been present for 1 month to 23 years (median, 15 months) at the time of diagnosis. They can begin either acutely or gradually: Both types of onset are equally common. Once started, symptoms worsen progressively. The progression can be either gradual (55% of cases) or stepwise with sudden deteriorations that improve only partially between attacks (45% of cases). In patients with stepwise deterioration and spinal cord involvement, multiple sclerosis is suggested. With stepwise deterioration and brain involvement, meningovascular syphilis and other forms of cerebral vascular disease are simulated.

Accompanying signs and symptoms of extraneural disease are present in fewer than 5% of patients. However, occasional patients have had fatigue, weight loss, fever, malaise, lymphadenopathy, backache, myalgia, or arthritis. In addition, retarded growth and sexual development were seen in two teenagers whose disease began in childhood, one of whom also had kyphosis.[6]

ENCEPHALITIS

Cerebral abnormalities are present in about 60% of patients with progressive borrelia encephalomyelitis (Figure 8–1). There is almost always (90%) an accompanying pleocytosis and, frequently, cranial neuritis (47%) or myelitis (30%). Accompanying radiculoneuritis is rare (6%).

The encephalopathy is focal or multifocal in 70% of cases, diffuse in 58%, and both diffuse and focal or multifocal in 24%. Sudden focal deficits, either permanent or transient, occur in 30% of those with cerebral symptoms. The most common focal abnormalities are hemiparesis (present in 15% of cases overall)[6,10,15,19,20,34–37] and dysphasia (12%)[d] (Figure 8–2), either of which may be transient. Dysarthria (21%)[6,10,15,23,26,34,36,38] and seizures (7%),[4–7,12,23,29]

---

[b]References 3, 11, 15, 18, 27, 28, 32, 35, 36, 38.
[c]References 6–8, 11, 13–15, 19, 20, 27, 30, 38.
[d]References 10, 11, 15, 19–21, 27, 34, 35, 37.

TYPE OF INVOLVEMENT

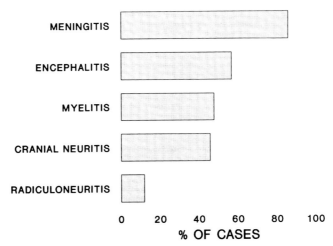

Figure 8–1. Frequency of major types of neurologic abnormalities in patients with progressive borrelia encephalomyelitis.

ABNORMALITY

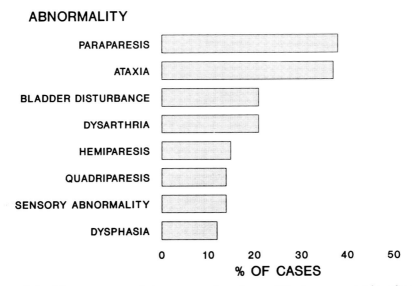

Figure 8–2. Most common central nervous system abnormalities in progressive borrelia encephalomyelitis.

both focal and generalized, are also relatively common, and paraparesis and quadriparesis occasionally are due to cerebral lesions, although they more often reflect spinal cord involvement. Typical signs and symptoms of more diffuse cerebral involvement, on which focal signs may be superimposed, include somnolence, confusion, poor concentration, restlessness and irritability, disorientation, and decreased memory. Occasional patients have had apraxia,[11] myoclonus,[10] hemiparesthesia,[24] visual field abnormalities,[19,20] alexia,[35] agraphia,[35] impairment of upward gaze,[15,35] and skew deviation[35] in addition.

Ataxia, particularly ataxia of gait, is also common (37% of cases), but it is not clear how often reported gait ataxia is caused by spasticity and sensory loss in the legs due to myelopathy and how often it is caused by cerebellar involvement alone. In some cases the cerebellum is definitely involved, as ataxia of all four limbs,[38] intention tremor in the arms,[6,11,15,26,34] and hemiataxia[24,35] have all been reported also.

The EEG in patients with cerebral involvement can be normal, slow, or dysrhythmic.[6] Reported abnormalities include focal slowing[11,15]; generalized slowing,[20] sometimes paroxysmal[12]; and bitemporal dysrhythmia with sharp waves.[23] CT has shown infarcts in the thalamus, internal capsule, and frontal and parietal lobes[12,26–28]; multiple hypodense foci in the cerebral white matter and periventricular areas,[6,19,20,24,37,38] sometimes with contrast enhancement[37,38]; hydrocephalus[19–21]; and cerebral atrophy with calcifications.[10] Similarly, MRI has demonstrated multiple hyperintense lesions in the periventricular white matter of the hemispheres and the brain stem (Figure 8–3)[e]; infarcts in the thalamus (Figure 8–4)[26]; ventricular enlargement[10]; paraventricular and insular cavities[10]; atrophy of the pons, medulla, and cervical spinal cord[10]; and diffuse increase in signal in the brain stem and cervical spinal cord.[7]

Moreover, in a number of cases, angiography has indicated cerebral vasculitis (Figure 8–5).[12,27,35,36] Reported abnormalities include irregularity of small and moderate-size vessels with narrowing, beading, multiple stenoses, and poststenotic dilatations; obstruction of branches of the middle and anterior cerebral arteries; and irregularity and occlusion of the basilar artery.

The prognosis in patients with cerebral involvement is not good. Symptoms do not resolve spontaneously, and, even with antibiotic treatment, residual disability is common. Occasional patients do recover completely, but most recover partially at best. In long-standing cases, a halt in the progression of the illness may be the only effect of treatment.

MYELITIS

The spinal cord is involved in about 50% of patients (see Figure 8–1). Accompanying pleocytosis is usual (95% of cases), and cerebral (60%) and cranial nerve (40%) involvement are common, but radiculoneuritis is rare (6%).

---

[e]References 6, 15, 17, 19, 20, 24, 25, 30, 38.

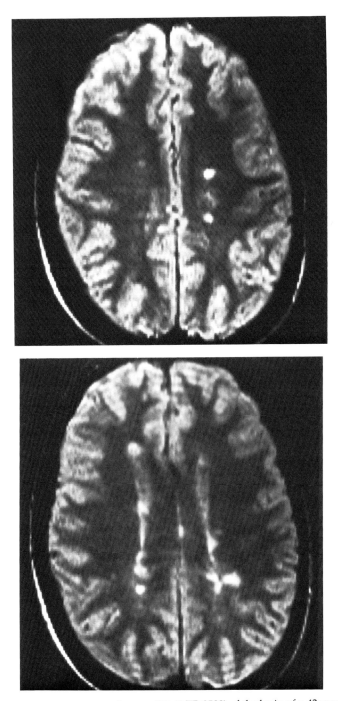

Figure 8–3. Magnetic resonance images (TE 40/TR 3500) of the brain of a 42-year-old woman with progressive borrelia encephalomyelitis of 2 years' duration that began 1 year after erythema migrans. There are multiple paraventricular areas of increased signal in the cerebral white matter.

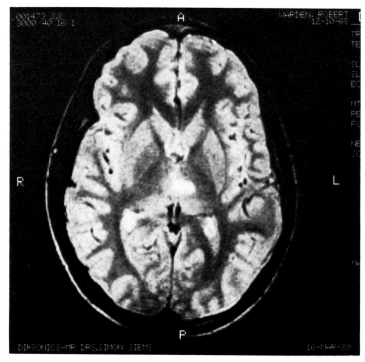

A

Figure 8–4. Magnetic resonance image of the brain of a 20-year-old man with progressive borrelia encephalomyelitis and stroke. *A.* Balanced T1/T2-weighted image shows an area of increased signal in the left thalamus. (Figure continued on next page.)

Myelitis most commonly presents with progressive spastic paraparesis or quadriparesis, which is severe in two-thirds of cases (see Figure 8–2). Associated urinary bladder abnormalities are common (33%), impotence and fecal incontinence less so. Sensory loss, usually mild, is less frequent (30%) than motor weakness. However, transverse myelitis with severe sensory loss has been reported in several cases with sensory levels at T_5, T_{11}, T_{12}, and L_4.[4,5,6,30]

Myelography is usually normal but did show arachnoiditis in one patient,[20] while MRI has demonstrated focal (Figure 8–6) or diffuse increase in signal intensity in the cervical spinal cord.[7] In at least three patients, somatosensory-evoked potentials have been abnormal.[9,15,17]

As is the case with cerebral involvement in chronic progressive borrelia encephalomyelitis, the outcome is often unfavorable, even with appropriate antibiotic therapy. Residual paresis and urinary abnormalities are common.

CRANIAL NEURITIS

Cranial nerve abnormalities are present in about 45% of patients, typically accompanied by pleocytosis (95%) and, less often, by cerebral abnormalities (50%) or myelitis (30%). Radiculitis is less usual (15%).

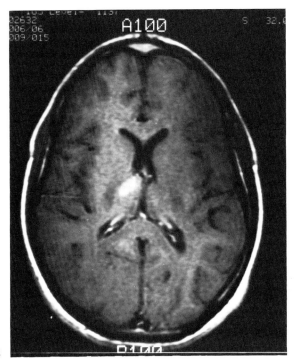

B

Figure 8–4, cont. *B.* T1-weighted, gadolinium-enhanced scan 1 month later shows an enhancing lesion in the right thalamus. (Reproduced from May EF, Jabbari B. *Stroke* 1990;21:1232–1235 by permission of the American Heart Association, Inc.)

The most common cranial nerve deficits are facial palsy (usually unilateral) and hearing loss (usually bilateral) (Figure 8–7).[6] Optic nerve involvement—optic neuritis, perineuritis, and papilledema—is slightly less common.[6,14,19,20,29,36] Involvement of cranial nerves III,[6] V,[37] and VI,[15,37] the vestibular portion of VIII,[30] IX,[6,37] X,[33] and XII[6,10] also has been reported in a few patients each.

Visual-evoked responses in several patients with optic nerve involvement have been abnormal,[14,15,20] and the brain stem auditory-evoked potential (BAER) in one patient with bilateral hearing loss showed a retrocochlear abnormality.[9]

As with the CNS abnormalities in progressive borrelia encephalomyelitis, residual cranial nerve deficit after treatment is common, particularly permanent hearing loss and optic atrophy, but recovery can take place.

RADICULONEURITIS

Radiculoneuritis is the least common neurologic abnormality in progressive borrelia encephalomyelitis, occurring in only 8% of patients.[6–8,23,30,37] Pleocytosis accompanies radiculoneuritis in only 50% of cases, and cerebral involvement, myelitis, and cranial neuritis are present in 50, 25, and 40%,

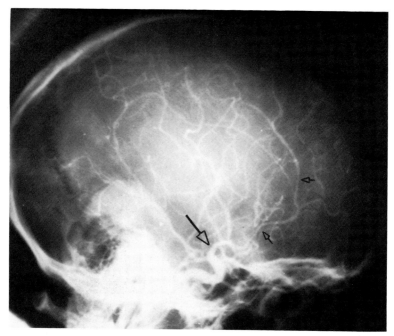

Figure 8–5. Carotid angiogram of a 22-year-old woman with Lyme disease and chronic meningitis, papilledema, and multiple episodes of transient left cheiro-oral numbness. The supraclinoid carotid artery is markedly narrowed (*large arrow*), and there are multiple other areas of arterial narrowing (*small arrows*) and dilatation consistent with vasculitis. (Courtesy of Dr. Arnold Witte, Trenton, NJ.)

respectively. In a few cases, progressive radiculoneuritis or meningoradiculitis, lasting 15 months to 8 years, has occurred without other nervous system involvement.[3,4,18,27,38] These cases, particularly those without pleocytosis, are probably more closely related to the other late peripheral neuropathies discussed later in this chapter.

Reported clinical patterns in patients with progressive borrelia encephalomyelitis and radiculoneuritis have included polyneuritis, mononeuritis simplex and multiplex, and radiculitis and radiculoplexitis.[6–8,23,30,37]

The outcome is often better in patients with peripheral than those with CNS deficits. Weakness frequently resolves in months after treatment, although persistent weakness can occur.

MENINGITIS

Pleocytosis, the most common abnormality in progressive borrelia encephalomyelitis, is present in 85% of patients (Table 8–1). But it is seldom symptomatic. Headache is reported in only 6% of patients, and neck stiffness in only 2%. Patients with pure radiculoneuritis or stroke are those most likely not to have pleocytosis.

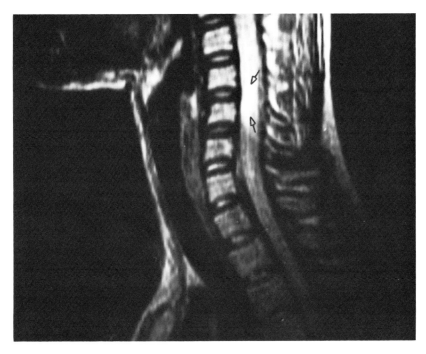

Figure 8–6. Magnetic resonance image (spin echo, TE 56/TR 1700) of the cervical spinal cord of a 33-year-old woman with stage 3 Lyme disease and cervical myelitis beginning 1 year after arthritis of the knees. There is an intramedullary area of increased signal intensity (*arrows*) at the C-5 level.

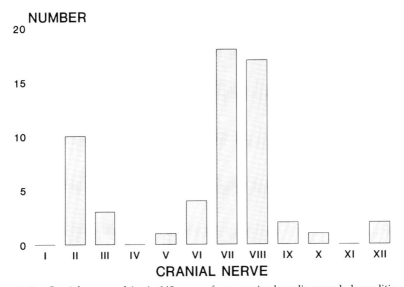

Figure 8–7. Cranial nerve palsies in 140 cases of progressive borrelia encephalomyelitis.

Table 8–1. CFS Findings in Progressive Borrelia Encephalomyelitis

Cell count	Elevated in 85%
Range	5–2300/mm³ (usually 100–200)
Lymphocytes (%)	> 90 in 95% of patients
Glucose	< 2/3 serum glucose in 10%
Protein	Up to 1800 mg/dL (usually 100–200)
Oligoclonal bands	Present in > 90% of patients
Increase in	
IgG	Present in > 90% of patients
IgA	Present in > 75% of patients
IgM	Present in > 75% of patients
Specific antibody	Present in > 95% of patients

The CSF pressure is only rarely increased. The fluid typically contains 100 to 200 cells/mm³ (up to 2300), usually lymphocytes (sometimes mixed with plasma cells[3,6,8,23,33,35–37]), but an excess of polymorphonuclear leukocytes (PMNs) is occasionally present.[8,20,36] In one patient, eosinophils were present in addition.[36] The protein is increased in 95% of patients, usually to 100 to 200 mg/dL (up to 1800). CSF IgG is almost always increased, and IgA and IgM usually so, while oligoclonal bands of IgG are present in over 90% of patients. The glucose level is usually normal, but it is decreased in as many as 10% of patients, sometimes as low as 12 mg/dL.[9,24] Almost all reported patients have had anti–*B. burgdorferi* antibody in both serum and CSF with evidence for intrathecal antibody synthesis. In a few patients, antibody was present in CSF but not in serum.[27,33] In a few others, particularly those from North America, measurable antibody was present only in serum.[30]

Pleocytosis usually subsides quickly after treatment, and cell counts are typically normal by 3 months, although minimal elevations can persist as long as a year. The CSF protein falls more slowly but is usually normal by 6 months. Anti–*B. burgdorferi* antibody may still be present in CSF as long as 5 years after successful treatment.[37]

Late Encephalopathy in North American Lyme Disease

The grave neurologic abnormalities of progressive borrelia encephalomyelitis are not frequent among North American patients with late Lyme disease, but milder yet nonetheless disabling CNS symptoms are. These symptoms have been delineated in most detail by Halperin and colleagues.[39,40] They pointed out that many patients with chronic Lyme disease have an antibiotic-responsive encephalitis characterized by defects in memory and concentration, accompanied often by profound fatigue but usually not by either physical abnormalities on neurologic examination or CSF inflammation.

In their first report,[39] Halperin et al. described 17 patients (average age, 39.2 years) with late Lyme disease (mean disease duration, 32.6 months) with defects in memory and cognition. A battery of neuropsychological tests,[f] administered to each of them, revealed readily identifiable and quantifiable deficits that correlated well with the patients' own perceptions of their disabilities. The abnormalities detected included defects in immediate and delayed auditory-verbal and visual memory, the ability to learn and retrieve new information, sustained attention and concentration, perceptual-motor performance, problem solving, and conceptual flexibility. The test scores improved significantly when the patients were retested 5 to 28 weeks after antibiotic treatment.

Other neurologic abnormalities were uncommon. None of the 17 patients had CNS abnormalities on examination, while only 4 had cranial or peripheral radiculopathy or neuropathy, only 2 had pleocytosis, and only 2 had EEG slowing. MRI, on the other hand, was abnormal in 4 of the 5 with the most severe subjective intellectual deficits, showing punctate hyperresonant areas in the cerebral white matter that were dense on both T1- and T2-weighted images (Figure 8–8).

In a second report,[40] the same authors described 22 patients with late disease and subjective changes in memory and cognition plus corresponding abnormalities on bedside mental status examination. Their median age was 34 years (range, 7 to 59 years) and the duration of their neurologic symptoms was 1 week to 8 years (median, 12 months). Twenty of them had had previous systemic symptoms compatible with Lyme disease: EM in 8 patients, a flu-like illness in 4, and arthralgias or arthritis in 16.

Anti–*B. burgdorferi* antibody was present in serum from 19 patients; T-cell assays were positive in the other 3. None had oligoclonal bands in the CSF, and the CSF IgG index was normal in all those tested. But 9 of 13 patients tested had intrathecal concentration of specific antibody, and 7 of 17 had white matter lesions on MRI that were hyperintense on T2- and proton-weighted images but isointense on T1-weighted images. Following treatment with intravenous ceftriaxone or penicillin, 18 patients improved clinically while the MRI abnormalities resolved in 3 of 6 after 3 to 10 months.

Similar findings were described by Logigian et al.[25] in 27 patients with immunoreactivity to *B. burgdorferi* who had had previous symptoms of Lyme disease and then developed neurologic symptoms without other cause months to years later. The neurologic symptoms began 1 month to 14 years after illness onset and had lasted 3 months to 14 years when the patients were examined. Twenty-four had encephalopathy characterized by defects in memory, mood changes (depression, irritability), sleep disorders, and word finding difficulties. Fourteen of the 24 had memory impairment on neuropsychologic tests, 11 had increased CSF protein, 11 had intrathecal production

---

[f]The tests included the California Verbal Learning Test, the Wechsler Memory Scale, the Information and Block Design subtests from the revised Wechsler Adult Intelligence Scale, the Symbol Digit Modalities Test, Trailmaking Tests parts A and B, the booklet version of the Categories Test, the Purdue Pegboard, and the Beck Depression Inventory.

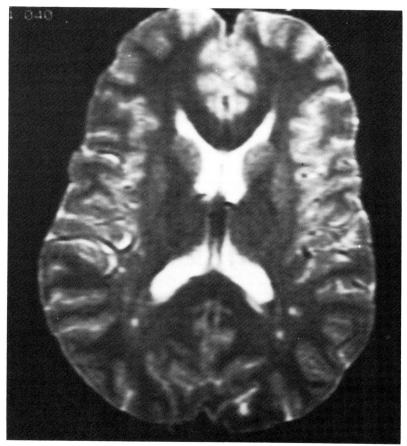

Figure 8–8.   Magnetic resonance image (TE 80/TR 2500) of the brain of a 32-year-old man with late Lyme disease and encephalopathy shows three punctate areas of increased signal intensity in the white matter adjacent to the posterior horns of the lateral ventricles. (Reproduced with permission from Reik L. In: Scheld WM, Whitley RJ, Durack DT, eds. *Infections of the Central Nervous System*. New York: Raven Press. In press.)

of anti–*B. burgdorferi* antibody, and 4 had white matter lesions on MRI. Concomitant polyneuropathy was present in 17 patients. Six months after treatment with intravenous ceftriaxone, 17 patients were improved, 6 had improved and then relapsed, and 4 were unchanged.

Children are affected also. The first report from Halperin et al.[39] included three children, and Pachner and Steere[29] described five others in whom neuropsychiatric symptoms developed months to years after the initial infection. These symptoms included difficulty concentrating, problems interacting with other children, mood swings, loss of friends, a decline in school performance, and, in one patient, an anorexia nervosa–like illness.

Specific antibody was present in the serum of all, but in the CSF of none. MRI was normal in the two patients tested.

Finally, Belman et al.[41] reported finding similar neurologic abnormalities in 38 seropositive children whose histories were compatible with late Lyme disease, although the disease duration was not specified. Headache (79% of patients) and behavioral change (42%)—irritability, emotional lability, worsening of attention deficit disorder, and decreased concentration and memory—were the most common abnormalities. School performance declined in 24%. Accompanying abnormalities included cranial neuropathy (16%), paresthesias (8%), peripheral neuropathy (8%), and focal motor deficits (3%). CSF pressure was increased in 20% (4 of 20) of those tested, 55% had either an increase in protein or pleocytosis of less than 50 cells/mm^3, 55% had anti–*B. burgdorferi* antibody in CSF, and 80% had detectable CSF immune complexes.

In sum, these several reports indicate that a mild antibiotic-responsive encephalitis is common among North American patients with late Lyme disease. They also suggest that reported cases of more severe CNS disease may represent only the most extreme examples of the same process.[39] But it is not clear whether this encephalitis results directly from CNS infection or indirectly through immunologic mechanisms.

Moreover, in a more recent study of 84 patients with a mild confusional state evaluated for presumed CNS Lyme disease, Halperin et al. suggested that the symptoms of many of these patients may be due to an encephalopathy, caused by the indirect toxic or metabolic effects of systemic infection, instead of an actual encephalitis.[42] They suggested this because 10 of the 14 immunopositive patients with cognitive dysfunction on bedside mental status testing whose CSF was examined did not have intrathecal antibody production, and only 21 of the 38 seropositive patients treated with antibiotics improved substantially. On the other hand, 4 of 5 patients with intrathecal antibody synthesis did respond to treatment. It is by no means certain, however, that the failure to detect intrathecal antibody production rules out CNS infection, and the exact cause of CNS symptoms in those patients without intrathecal synthesis remains to be determined.

Other Central Nervous System Abnormalities

LYME DISEASE AND MULTIPLE SCLEROSIS

A number of authors have noted the similarity in neurologic appearance and course of CNS Lyme disease and multiple sclerosis (MS) and the possibility of mistaking one for the other.[5,6,19,30,43–47] Chronic progressive encephalomyelitis, especially the predominantly spinal form, can be confused clinically with MS because of its sometimes remitting and relapsing course and the high incidence of spinal motor signs, ataxia, bladder dysfunction, and, less often, optic neuritis.[5,6] Acute transverse myelitis, when it develops in stage 2 Lyme disease, may also cause diagnostic confusion.[47] Adding to the similarity between the two illnesses are the presence of oligoclonal bands of IgG and increased levels of IgG in the CSF in most patients with severe CNS Lyme disease, and the presence of periventricular white matter lesions on CT and MRI in many. But severe CNS Lyme disease can usually be distinguished from MS by the presence of a more brisk pleocytosis and more marked blood-brain barrier dysfunction, while an additional clue in some patients is the simultaneous presence of peripheral nervous system abnormalities.

Because of the similarities between the two illnesses, some speculation about a causal role for *B. burgdorferi* or related organisms in MS was inevitable.[48-50] A number of studies have now shown, however, that the frequency of serum antibodies against *B. burgdorferi* is no higher among patients with MS from areas endemic for Lyme disease than it is among normal controls from the same region.[20,51-53] In addition, patients with clinically definite MS and specific antibody in serum do not show evidence of intrathecal synthesis of the antibody.[40] It seems unlikely, therefore, that there is any causal relationship between *B. burgdorferi* infection and the development of MS: MS patients who are seropositive probably have had only coincidental exposure to the organism.

LYME DISEASE AND MOTOR NEURON DISEASE

A possible relationship between Lyme disease and motor neuron disease was first suggested when 4 of 54 patients from Wisconsin and Illinois with amyotrophic lateral sclerosis (ALS) were found to have significant titers of anti–*B. burgdorferi* antibody in serum, and one of them appeared to stabilize clinically after antibiotic therapy.[54]

In response to this report and the publicity it received, Mandell et al. examined serum from 71 patients with ALS who were followed in Boston.[55] Nine patients had slightly increased antibody responses to *B. burgdorferi* (IgG in 3, IgM in 6), but immunoblots from only 3 of the 9 showed specific antibody bands, and these were only weak IgM bands reacting with the organism's 60- and 66-kd proteins. The authors concluded that they could not confirm that *B. burgdorferi* is an etiologic agent of ALS.

A subsequent epidemiologic study from Long Island, New York, however, again suggested a relationship between *B. burgdorferi* infection and ALS.[56] Nine (47%) of 19 ALS patients from Suffolk County, a hyperendemic area for Lyme disease, were seropositive and immunoblot reactive against the organism, and 3 of them improved following antibiotic therapy. Moreover, serum antibody was present in only 3 of 14 ALS patients from adjacent, but less rural, Nassau County; in only 4 of 38 matched controls from these areas; and in only 1 of 19 ALS patients followed at the Massachusetts General Hospital in Boston.

The clinical findings in seropositive patients did not differ significantly from those in seronegative patients, and all appeared to have typical ALS.

Laboratory findings were also not significantly different: only 1 of 21 immuno-reactive patients had CSF pleocytosis (8 cells/mm³); 6 had increased protein (range, 48 to 148 mg/dL); and 3, all of whom had severe bulbar dysfunction, had intrathecal antibody synthesis. Electromyographic findings were typical of ALS, showing acute and chronic denervation and fasciculations in all patients.

The electroneurographic findings were not as typical, however, with some abnormality recorded in 9 of 21 immunoreactive patients. In 5 of 6 patients tested, the amplitude of the compound muscle action potential was markedly decreased, but not dispersed, following stimulation at Erb's point; 3 patients had prolongation of the F response; 2 patients had delayed H reflexes; and 4 had mononeuropathy or slowing of motor nerve conduction velocity (NCV) to below 40 m/sec in a single nerve. Among 11 immunonega-tive ALS patients, only 1 had a prolonged F response, and only 1 slowing of motor NCV below 40 m/sec.

The authors concluded that only the 3 patients with severe bulbar involvement and intrathecal antibody synthesis had CNS *B. burgdorferi* infec-tion. The others, they suggested, may have suffered from a *B. burgdorferi*–associated motor polyneuropathy that caused a clinical picture similar to ALS with mainly lower motor neuron involvement.

It does appear that Lyme disease can mimic ALS, therefore; but how often it does so is not clear. If it does so frequently, then the incidence of ALS should be higher in endemic areas.

LATENT CENTRAL NERVOUS SYSTEM DISEASE

Ackermann et al.[6] described four patients who they believe had latent CNS infection with *B. burgdorferi*; three had had a spontaneously resolving stage 2 meningopolyneuritis 3, 6, and 12 years earlier. One of the four had a slight residual facial palsy, one had a loss of Achilles reflexes, and one had migrating pains without clinical signs. All four had intrathecally synthesized anti–*B. burgdorferi* antibody without pleocytosis, increase in CSF protein, or elevated CSF IgG content.

While it is clear that latent CNS infection with *B. burgdorferi* does occur—the organism has been cultured from normal CSF[1] and late CNS abnor-malities can develop long after the initial infection (*vide supra*)—it is also clear that the presence of specific antibody in the CSF is not sufficient evidence to prove latent infection. Antibody can persist in the CSF as long as 5 years after the successful treatment of progressive borrelia encephalomyelitis[37] and as long as 21 years after spontaneously resolving meningopolyneuritis.[52] In-deed, Krüger et al.[52] found that 11 of 27 untreated meningopolyneuritis patients reexamined 5 to 21 years after resolution had positive borrelia-specific immunoblots in the CSF, even though none had experienced any progression of symptoms.

It seems likely, therefore, that the persistence of specific anti–*B. burgdor-*

feri antibody in the CSF is not a measure of either persistence or latency but merely a reflection of previous CNS infection. A reliable indicator of latent infection remains to be determined.

Peripheral Nervous System Abnormalities

Distal Axonopathy

In a series of reports comprising 164 North American patients with Lyme disease, Halperin et al. described a multifocal polyneuropathy that is milder than stage 2 meningopolyneuritis, with less dramatic signs and symptoms, and does not improve spontaneously.[39,57,58] About 25% of those affected have accompanying mild cerebral symptoms, but signs of CNS involvement are seldom present.

As many as 50% of these authors' patients with late Lyme disease (defined by them as disease of ≥ 4 weeks' duration) have tingling paresthesias of the extremities.[39,57,58] These usually begin months after illness onset (median, 6 months; mean, 22.5 months), and typically have been present a year or more at the time of clinical evaluation (median, 12 months; mean, 27.4 months).[58] The paresthesias are often intermittent; can involve the arms, the legs, or both; and are commonly distal but can be patchy in distribution. About 25% of patients with paresthesias have a mild stocking/glove distal sensory loss, but motor weakness and reflex loss are rare.

Radicular pain is less common, occurring in about 25% of patients with late disease.[39,57,58] It also begins months after illness onset (median, 5 months; mean, 16.8 months), but its presence prompts evaluation sooner than paresthesias do (median, 9 months; mean, 17 months).[58] The legs are most often the site of the pain (75%), the arms (20%) and the trunk (5%) less often so.[58] The location of the pain is not consistently related to the site of the initial tick bite.[58]

The carpal tunnel syndrome (CTS) also develops in about 25% of patients with late disease (disease duration, 4 months to 9 years; mean, 37 months).[39,57–59] Affected patients typically have intermittent paresthesias in the median nerve distribution that are exacerbated during sleep or by use of the hands. Symptoms are bilateral in two-thirds. There is usually no accompanying wrist tenosynovitis or arthritis. Accompanying motor weakness is seldom present.

Electrophysiologic testing has shown abnormalities of two or more peripheral nerves in 40 to 50% of patients with late disease, including some without symptoms.[39,57,58] The most common abnormalities, typically multifocal, are slowing of sensory NCV or decreased sensory amplitude or both (52% of patients); prolongation of distal motor latency, slowing of motor NCV, or decreased compound action potential (40%); and increased F wave latency (40%). Halperin et al. interpret these abnormalities as indicating a patchy, mainly distal, axonal neuropathy and suggest that it results from a vasculopathy.[39,57,58] However, demyelination can occur also, although rarely: At least one patient has had severe slowing of conduction velocity and multiple areas of conduction block.

Patients with electrophysiologic evidence for CTS have slowing of segmental conduction (100%), slowing of sensory (70%) or motor NCV (65%) across the wrist, and decreased sensory amplitude (14%) in the median nerve. In 43% of cases the abnormalities are bilateral.[59]

Other laboratory abnormalities are uncommon. In one series, however, three of seven patients tested did have pleocytosis and increased CSF protein without increased IgG or oligoclonal bands.[57]

Paresthesias almost always improve, as do the accompanying electrophysiologic abnormalities, within 3 to 7 months after antibiotic (ceftriaxone) therapy. Radicular pain and symptoms of CTS, on the other hand, each improve in only about 50% of patients following treatment.

Neuropathy in Acrodermatitis Chronica Atrophicans

Peripheral neuropathy is common also among European patients with ACA, 25 to 70% of whom have neuropathic symptoms.[60–64] The symptoms are usually asymmetric and most marked in the area of the skin lesion.[60,63,64] They include paresthesias, burning dysesthesias, sharp pains, hyperesthesia, weakness, and muscle cramps.

Characteristic physical signs, present in up to 65%, are reflex changes (7 to 40%); hypesthesia and hypalgesia (25%), especially in areas of skin atrophy; impaired vibratory sense (20%); muscle weakness (15%) and atrophy (5%); and hyperpathia (5%).[60,63,64] The signs, like the symptoms, are usually asymmetric and most marked in regions of skin involvement. Several clinical patterns result, including cutaneous mononeuropathy, distal asymmetric polyneuropathy, and distal symmetric polyneuropathy.[63] In one unusual case, a typical Guillain-Barré syndrome began 22 months after the onset of ACA and appeared to respond to penicillin therapy.[65]

Systemic signs and symptoms may accompany ACA-associated neuropathy.[62] Those most common are profound fatigue, lymphadenopathy, subluxation of small joints in the hands and feet, and intermittent arthritis of the knee. Accompanying personality change has also been reported,[62] but physical signs of CNS disease are usually not present. However, CNS involvement may occur: One-third of 26 patients with ACA in one report had abnormal BAERs which returned to normal after antibiotic treatment.[62]

Electrophysiologic abnormalities are present in most symptomatic patients and up to 25% of those without symptoms.[60,63,64] The abnormalities reported resemble those recorded from North American patients with late Lyme disease and distal axonopathy. Motor and sensory NCVs are mildly slowed in most cases, while the distal latencies are prolonged and the compound action potentials dispersed with decreased amplitude in many. Yet at least two reported patients have had very slow NCVs (21 and 22 m/sec) indicating demyelination.[63]

Neuropathic symptoms and signs accompanying ACA generally improve with antibiotic therapy. The frequency of clinical neuropathy is lower (28%) among patients who are first examined neurologically after treatment than among those who are untreated (62%).[63] The symptoms of some patients, but not others, have improved even with low-dose oral penicillin therapy (4 million units/day for 2 weeks).[60] The response of the electrophysiologic abnormalities to therapy has not been reported, however.

Neuropathy with Other Late Sclerotic Skin Lesions

In a recent study, Aberer et al.[66] evaluated the nervous system of nine patients with morphea and two with lichen sclerosus et atrophica (LSA), most of whom had evidence for *B. burgdorferi* infection. There were ten women and one man, aged 21 to 83 years (median, 48), whose disease duration was 1 month to 26 years (median, 2 years). Six patients had anti–*B. burgdorferi* antibody in serum, and lesional biopsy specimens from four (three with morphea, one with LSA), including two who were seronegative, revealed spirochetes when stained with an avidin-biotin-immunoperoxidase technique. In addition, *Borrelia* were cultured from a biopsy specimen of the skin lesion of one seropositive patient who had had morphea for 2 years.

The neurologic findings were similar to those seen in patients with ACA. Eight of the nine morphea patients and both LSA patients had lesional dysesthesias, hypoesthesia, hyperesthesia, or pain, suggesting degeneration of the free nerve endings in the area of the skin lesion. One patient with LSA had a symmetric sensorimotor polyneuropathy in the legs in addition. Other neurologic abnormalities included a previous facial palsy in one, and weakness and wasting of the thigh in one other.

Electrophysiologic tests showed prolongation of the distal motor latency of a single nerve in the extremity with the skin lesion in 2 patients with morphea. In one of these two, there were also myopathic changes in the quadriceps muscle. The compound action potentials of several nerves in the legs were reduced in amplitude in the patient with generalized extragenital LSA and sensorimotor polyneuropathy.

The CSF was abnormal in three of seven patients tested. The abnormalities detected included blood-brain barrier disruption in one, intrathecal synthesis of specific antibody in a second, and pleocytosis (27 cells/mm^3) and oligoclonal bands of IgG in a third.

After antibiotic therapy, the pleocytosis disappeared but the oligoclonal bands persisted. The response to treatment of the other laboratory abnormalities and of the neuropathic symptoms was not reported, however.

Myositis

Myositis has been reported in late (stage 3) Lyme disease, but it appears to be less common than and to differ histologically from the myositis of stage 2 disease. Reimers et al. described four such cases in patients with ACA and elevated serum levels of anti–*B. burgdorferi* antibody: Three had focal nodular myositis and the fourth, inclusion body myositis.[67] Two of these cases were reported in detail.[68]

The first patient, a 66-year-old woman with ACA of the left arm developed progressive weakness of multiple muscle groups in both legs over 4 months. The serum creatine kinase (CK) level was normal, but electrophysiologic tests revealed a mixture of neuropathic and myopathic abnormalities in the legs: slightly decreased motor NCV in the peroneal nerve; delayed, low-amplitude H waves; both low-amplitude, short-duration and high-amplitude, long-duration polyphasic potentials; and fibrillations and positive sharp waves. Muscle biopsy specimens showed focal perivascular round cell infiltration with adjacent areas of muscle fiber necrosis and degeneration (focal nodular myositis). Spirochetes were present in the muscle on silver stains. Eight months after treatment with intravenous penicillin and then oral minocycline, muscle strength had returned to normal, and the electromyographic abnormalities had disappeared.

The second patient, a 61-year-old man, had progressive ACA of the right leg, an absent right sural sensory potential, and positive sharp waves in the medial head of the right gastrocnemius. The serum CK level was elevated (201 units/L), and MRI demonstrated increased signal intensity in the medial right gastrocnemius on T2-weighted images. Gastrocnemius biopsy specimens revealed focal nodular myositis. Spirochetes were present on silver stained sections. Three months after intravenous cefotaxime and then ceftriaxone therapy, the MRI abnormalities had improved.

In one additional patient, not associated with ACA, a 58-year-old man developed progressive atrophy of both quadriceps muscles over an 8-year period following an EM and subsequent meningopolyneuritis.[27] Electrophysiologic testing indicated a peripheral neurogenic lesion, but a muscle biopsy specimen showed an inflammatory necrotizing myopathy. Two months after treatment with intravenous penicillin, examination showed a slight increase in muscular strength in the thighs.

Stage 3 Neuroborreliosis in Children

It should be no surprise that the nervous system abnormalities of late Lyme disease are less common in children than in adults. Since many of these abnormalities develop years after the initial infection, late neurologic complications of disease acquired in childhood may not appear until early adult life. ACA in particular is found predominantly in older individuals, and the neuropathy that accompanies ACA has not been described in children, nor has focal nodular myositis. However, late encephalopathy can begin in childhood,[29,39,41] as can progressive borrelia encephalomyelitis,[6,10] although both are more common in adults. Paresthesias and peripheral neuropathy have also been reported in childhood,[41] but the CTS has not.

European versus North American Late Lyme Disease

There are also some apparent contrasts between the neurologic abnormalities of late Lyme disease in Europe and North America. One obvious difference is that progressive borrelia encephalomyelitis is much more frequent in Europe than in North America, where only a few cases have been reported so far.[11,12,25,29,30] The syndrome is probably more frequent in Europe at present because progressive borrelia encephalomyelitis has a long incubation period and Lyme disease has been common in North America for a relatively short time. Whether strain differences are also a factor is not known, but with time and increased awareness, I expect more cases to be reported from North America.

ACA also appears to be almost uniquely European,[62] although a few cases have been reported from North America.[69] Yet its higher incidence in Europe, like that of progressive encephalomyelitis, may only reflect the longer history of Lyme disease there plus a greater familiarity with the skin lesion among European dermatologists. Since ACA is less common in North America, however, so is the neuropathy associated with it. But the distal axonopathy described by Halperin et al.[57,58] in North American patients with late Lyme disease does not appear to differ substantially from the neuropathy associated with ACA in clinical manifestations, electrophysiologic findings, and pathologic features; the two are probably manifestations of the same process. Whether a similar axonopathy occurs in European patients without ACA has not been studied to my knowledge.

A final major difference concerns the frequency of mild cerebral symptoms in North American patients with late Lyme disease. As with the similar mild cerebral symptoms in North American patients with stage 2 disease, it is not clear whether the apparent disparity is real and a reflection of genuine divergence between the organism and the disease it causes on the two continents, or whether cerebral symptoms of this type are equally frequent in Europe but have not been sought as systematically there.

References

1. Pfister H-W, Preac-Mursic V, Wilske B, Einhäupl K-M, Weinberger K. Latent Lyme neuroborreliosis: Presence of *Borrelia burgdorferi* in the cerebrospinal fluid without concurrent inflammatory signs. *Neurology* 1989;39:1118–1120.
2. Preac-Mursic V, Weber K, Pfister HW, et al. Survival of *Borrelia burgdorferi* in antibiotically treated patients with Lyme borreliosis. *Infection* 1989;17:355–359.
3. Wokke JHJ, de Koning J, Stanek G, Jennekens FGI. Chronic muscle weakness caused by *Borrelia burgdorferi* meningoradiculitis. *Ann Neurol* 1987;22:389–392.
4. Ackermann R, Gollmer E, Rehse-Küpper B. Progressive Borrelien-Enzephalomyelitis: chronische Manifestation der Erythema-chronicum-migrans-Krankheit am Nervensystem. *Dtsch Med Wochenschr* 1985;110:1039–1042.
5. Ackermann R, Rehse-Küpper B, Gollmer E. Progressive borrelia encephalomyelitis. *Zentralbl Bakteriol Mikrobiol Hyg [A]* 1986;263:297–300.

6. Ackermann R, Rehse-Küpper B, Gollmer E, Schmidt R. Chronic neurologic manifestations of erythema migrans borreliosis. *Ann NY Acad Sci* 1988;539:16–23.
7. Ackermann R. Tertiary neuroborreliosis: The enlarging spectrum. Presented at the Fourth International Conference on Lyme Borreliosis; June 18–21, 1990; Stockholm, Sweden.
8. Behringer A, Wirbatz A. Chronische Borrelien-Erkrankung des Zentralen Nervensystems. *Nervenarzt* 1987;58:564–567.
9. Benoit P, Dournon E, Masingue M, Destee A, Warot P. Méningonévraxite borrélienne: un cas. *Presse Med* 1987;16:1733–1736.
10. Bensch J, Olcén P, Hagberg L. Destructive chronic borrelia meningoencephalitis in a child untreated for 15 years. *Scand J Infect Dis* 1987;19:697–700.
11. Broderick JP, Sandok BA, Mertz LE. Focal encephalitis in a young woman 6 years after the onset of Lyme disease: Tertiary Lyme disease? *Mayo Clin Proc* 1987;62:313–316.
12. Brogan GX, Homan CS, Viccellio P. The enlarging clinical spectrum of Lyme disease: Lyme cerebral vasculitis, a new disease entity. *Ann Emerg Med* 1990;19:572–576.
13. Carlsson M, Malmvall B-E. Borrelia infection as a cause of presenile dementia. *Lancet* 1987;2:798.
14. Del Sette M, Caponnetto C, Fumarola D, Mancardi GL. Unusual neurological manifestations of Lyme disease: A case report. *Ital J Neurol Sci* 1989;10:455–456.
15. Depré A, Sindic CJM, Bukaska K, Bigaignon G, Laterre C. Formes encéphalomyélitiques de l'infection a *Borrelia burgdorferi*. *Rev Neurol (Paris)* 1988;144:416–420.
16. Fredrikson S, Link H. CNS-borreliosis selectively affecting central motor neurons. *Acta Neurol Scand* 1988;78:181–184.
17. Hänny PE, Häuselmann HJ. Die Lyme-Krankheit aus der Sicht des Neurologen. *Schweiz Med Wochenschr* 1987;117:901–915.
18. Klöter I, Adam T, Schabet M, Wiethölter, Peiffer J. Borrelia-induced meningoradiculitis—two different forms of the disease. *Eur Neurol* 1986;25:262–268.
19. Kohler J, Kasper J, Kern U, Thoden U, Rehse-Küpper B. Borrelia encephalomyelitis. *Lancet* 1986;2:35.
20. Kohler J, Kern U, Kasper J, Rehse-Küpper B, Thoden U. Chronic central nervous system involvement in Lyme borreliosis. *Neurology* 1988;38:863–867.
21. Kohlhepp W, Mertens H-G, Oschmann P. Acute and chronic illness after tick-bite *Borrelia burgdorferi*–infections: Results of treatment. *Zentralbl Bakteriol Mikrobiol Hyg [A]* 1986; 263:365–371.
22. Kohlhepp W, Mertens HG, Oschmann P, Rohrbach E. Akute und chronische Erkrankungen bei zeckenvermittelter Borreliose. *Nervenarzt* 1987;58:557–563.
23. Kollikowski HH, Schwendemann G, Schulz M, Wilhelm H, Lehmann H-J. Chronic borrelia encephalomyeloradiculitis with severe mental disturbance: Immunosuppressive versus antibiotic therapy. *J Neurol* 1988;235:140–142.
24. Lock G, Berger G, Gröbe H. Neuroborreliose: progressive Encephalomyelitis mit cerebraler Vaskulitis. *Monatsschr Kinderheilkd* 1989;137:101–104.
25. Logigian EL, Kaplan RF, Steere AC. Chronic neurologic manifestations of Lyme disease. *N Engl J Med* 1990;323:1438–1444.
26. May EF, Jabbari B. Stroke in neuroborreliosis. *Stroke* 1990;21:1232–1235.
27. Midgard R, Hofstad H. Unusual manifestations of nervous system *Borrelia burgdorferi* infection. *Arch Neurol* 1987;44:781–783.
28. Olsson J-E. Henriksson A, Johansson I. Neuroborreliosis as a cause of ischemic stroke. Presented at the Fourth International Conference on Lyme Borreliosis; June 18–21, 1990; Stockholm, Sweden.
29. Pachner AR, Steere AC. CNS manifestations of third stage Lyme disease. *Zentralbl Bakteriol Mikrobiol Hyg [A]* 1986;263:301–306.
30. Pachner AR, Duray P, Steere AC. Central nervous system manifestations of Lyme disease. *Arch Neurol* 1989;46:790–795.
31. Pfister H-W, Einhäupl KM, Wilske B, Preac-Mursic V. Bannwarth's syndrome and the enlarged neurological spectrum of arthropod-borne borreliosis. *Zentralbl Bakteriol Mikrobiol Hyg [A]* 1986;263:343–347.
32. Riedmann G, Barolin GS. Neuroborreliose. *Wien Med Wochenschr* 1988;138:613–616.
33. Ryberg B. Bannwarth's syndrome (lymphocytic meningoradiculitis) in Sweden. *Yale J Biol Med* 1984;57:499–503.
34. Sindic CJM, Depre A, Bigaignon G, Goubau PF, Hella P, Laterre C. Lymphocytic meningoradiculitis and encephalomyelitis due to *Borrelia burgdorferi*: A clinical and serological study of 18 cases. *J Neurol Neurosurg Psychiatry* 1987;50:1565–1571.

35. Uldry P-A, Regli F, Bogousslavsky J. Cerebral angiopathy and recurrent strokes following *Borrelia burgdorferi* infection. *J Neurol Neurosurg Psychiatry* 1987;50:1703–1704.
36. Veenendaal-Hilbers JA, Perquin WVM, Hoogland PH, Doornbos L. Basal meningovasculitis and occlusion of the basilar artery in two cases of *Borrelia burgdorferi* infection. *Neurology* 1988;38:1317–1319.
37. Weder B, Wiedersheim P, Matter L, Steck A, Otto F. Chronic progressive neurological involvement in *Borrelia burgdorferi* infection. *J Neurol* 1987;234:40–43.
38. Wokke JHJ, van Gijn J, Elderson A, Stanek G. Chronic forms of *Borrelia burgdorferi* infection of the nervous system. *Neurology* 1987;37:1031–1034.
39. Halperin JJ, Pass HL, Anand AK, Luft BJ, Volkman DJ, Dattwyler R. Nervous system abnormalities in Lyme disease. *Ann NY Acad Sci* 1988;539:24–34.
40. Halperin JJ, Luft BJ, Anand AK, et al. Lyme neuroborreliosis: Central nervous system manifestations. *Neurology* 1989;39:753–759.
41. Belman AL, Coyle PK, Schutzer SE, Engel M, Dattwyler R. Neurologic involvement in pediatric Lyme disease. *Ann Neurol* 1989;26:476.
42. Halperin JJ, Krupp LB, Golightly MG, Volkman DJ. Lyme-borreliosis-associated encephalopathy. *Neurology* 1990;40:1340–1343.
43. Baumhackl U, Kristoferitsch W, Sluga E, Stanek G. Neurological manifestations of *Borrelia burgdorferi*–infections: The enlarging clinical spectrum. *Zentralbl Bakteriol Mikrobiol Hyg [A]* 1986;263:334–336.
44. Benoit P, Dournon E, Destee A, Warot P. Spirochaetes and Lyme disease. *Lancet* 1986;2:1223.
45. Pachner AR. Spirochetal diseases of the CNS. *Neurol Clin* 1986;4:207–222.
46. Pachner AR. *Borrelia burgdorferi* in the nervous system: The new "great imitator". *Ann NY Acad Sci* 1988;539:56–64.
47. Rousseau JJ, Lust C, Zangerle PF, Bigaignon G. Acute transverse myelitis as presenting neurological feature of Lyme disease. *Lancet* 1986;2:1222–1223.
48. Gay D, Dick G. Is multiple sclerosis caused by an oral spirochaete? *Lancet* 1986;2:75–77.
49. Marshall V. Letter to the editor. *J Neurol Sci* 1988;84:117–118.
50. Kurtz SK. Relapsing fever/Lyme disease/multiple sclerosis. *Med Hypotheses* 1986;3:335–343.
51. Coyle PK. *Borrelia burgdorferi* antibodies in multiple sclerosis patients. *Neurology* 1989;39:760–761.
52. Krüger H, Reuss K, Pulz M, et al. Meningoradiculitis and encephalomyelitis due to *Borrelia burgdorferi*: A follow-up study of 72 patients over 27 years. *J Neurol* 1989;236:322–328.
53. Schmutzhard E, Pohl P, Stanek G. *Borrelia burgdorferi* antibodies in patients with relapsing/remitting form and chronic progressive form of multiple sclerosis. *J Neurol Neurosurg Psychiatry* 1988;51:1215–1218.
54. Waisbren BA, Cashman N, Schell RF, Johnson R. *Borrelia burgdorferi* antibodies and amyotrophic lateral sclerosis. *Lancet* 1987;2:332–333.
55. Mandell H, Steere AC, Reinhardt BN, et al. Lack of antibodies to *Borrelia burgdorferi* in patients with amyotrophic lateral sclerosis. *N Engl J Med* 1989;320:255–256.
56. Halperin JJ, Kaplan GP, Brazinsky S, et al. Immunologic reactivity against *Borrelia burgdorferi* in patients with motor neuron disease. *Arch Neurol* 1990;47:586–594.
57. Halperin JJ, Little BW, Coyle PK, Dattwyler RJ. Lyme disease: Cause of a treatable peripheral neuropathy. *Neurology* 1987;37:1700–1706.
58. Halperin J, Luft BJ, Volkman DJ, Dattwyler RJ. Lyme neuroborreliosis: Peripheral nervous system manifestations. *Brain* 1990;113:1207–1221.
59. Halperin JJ, Volkman DJ, Luft BJ, Dattwyler RJ. Carpal tunnel syndrome in Lyme borreliosis. *Muscle Nerve* 1989;12:397–400.
60. Hopf HC. Peripheral neuropathy in acrodermatitis chronica atrophicans (Herxheimer). *J Neurol Neurosurg Psychiatry* 1975;38:452–458.
61. Burgdorf WHC, Worret W-I, Schultka O. Acrodermatitis chronica atrophicans. *Int J Dermatol* 1979;18:596–601.
62. Åsbrink E, Hovmark A. Early and late cutaneous manifestations in *Ixodes*-borne borreliosis (erythema migrans borreliosis, Lyme borreliosis). *Ann NY Acad Sci* 1988;539:4–15.
63. Kristoferitsch W, Sluga E, Graf M, et al. Neuropathy associated with acrodermatitis chronica atrophicans: Clinical and morphological features. *Ann NY Acad Sci* 1988;539:35–45.
64. Kindstrand E, Åsbrink E, Nilsson BY, Hovmark A. Peripheral neuropathy in chronic borrelia infection. Presented at the Fourth International Conference on Lyme Borreliosis; June 18–21, 1990; Stockholm, Sweden.

65. Goor W, Ott F. Zirkulationsstörung—Acrodermatitis chronica atrophicans Pick-Herxheimer? *Schweiz Med Wochenschr* 1971;101:1334–1338.
66. Aberer E, Kollegger H, Kristoferitsch W, Stanek G. Neuroborreliosis in morphea and lichen sclerosus et atrophicus. *J Am Acad Dermatol* 1988;19:820–825.
67. Reimers CD, de Koning J, Pilz A, et al. Myositis associated with *Borrelia burgdorferi*–infection. Presented at the Fourth International Conference on Lyme Borreliosis; June 18–21, 1990; Stockholm, Sweden.
68. Reimers CD, Pongratz DE, Neubert U, et al. Myositis caused by *Borrelia burgdorferi*: Report of four cases. *J Neurol Sci* 1989;91:215–226.
69. Lavoie PE, Wilson AJ, Tuffanelli DL. Acrodermatitis chronica atrophicans with antecedent Lyme disease in a Californian. *Zentralbl Bakteriol Mikrobiol Hyg [A]* 1986;263:262–265.

9

Diagnosis of Nervous System Lyme Disease

Laboratory Diagnosis

The laboratory diagnosis of Lyme disease is usually made serologically since the isolation of *Borrelia burgdorferi* from patients is difficult, and the small number of organisms in infected tissues precludes their routine identification in stained sections of specimens.

While other methods of demonstrating *Borrelia burgdorferi* antigens and genetic material in fluids and tissues of patients are being developed and do show promise, none is yet available for regular clinical use. Monoclonal antibodies have been used to demonstrate specific antigen in urine from infected mice and humans,[1] but the accuracy of the test is not known and its clinical usefulness remains to be demonstrated.[2] Other recent investigations have focused on the creation of DNA probes[3] and the use of the polymerase chain reaction[4] to identify the *B. burgdorferi* genome, but these techniques have been applied to few patient specimens thus far and they too remain experimental.

In some cases, nonspecific laboratory tests can provide a diagnostic clue—in patients with stage 2 neurologic involvement, at least in North America, the ESR is often elevated, serum IgM may be increased, and serum may contain cryoimmunoglobulins, their levels often paralleling disease activity—but routine laboratory test results are usually otherwise normal.[5] In late cases, even these few abnormalities are typically absent. Consequently, the laboratory diagnosis of Lyme disease is usually based on demonstrating an immune response to *B. burgdorferi*.

Antibody Tests

SERUM ANTIBODY TESTS

The presence of specific antibody *B. burgdorferi* is the best laboratory indication of Lyme disease, and a positive test result in a patient with compatible neurologic abnormalities is strong evidence for the diagnosis.

Anti–*B. burgdorferi* antibodies can be assayed by both indirect immunofluorescent (IFA) and by enzyme-linked immunosorbent assays (ELISA).[6–11] Although both techniques give similar results, the ELISA is preferred at present as it is more specific and more sensitive.[6,9–12] The ELISA is also more easily standardized and automated, and its absorbance values can be statistically analyzed, while interpretation of the IFA is more subjective.

When the ELISA technique is used, IgM and IgG usually are measured separately. Serum IgM antibody appears first, but it is often not present when erythema migrans (EM) begins. Raised IgM levels usually appear 2 to 4 weeks after the start of infection, with the antibodies directed mainly against the 41-kd flagellar antigen. The antibody levels typically peak at 6 to 8 weeks, and then gradually decline, although IgM antibodies occasionally persist throughout the course of infection.[6,8,10,13,14]

IgG antibody appears later. The levels are not raised during the first 4 to 6 weeks of infection but become elevated during the second and third months.[6,8,10,13,14] Once the levels of IgG antibody are raised, they can remain so for years, even after successful treatment or during clinical remission. If the disease remains active, the antibody response expands with time to include IgG and even IgM antibodies against additional antigens, particularly outer surface proteins (osp) A and B, and protein C (pC).[14] Serum levels of specific IgA antibody, whose rise parallels that of IgG,[15] are not measured routinely.

By the time neurologic symptoms appear in stage 2, therefore, serum levels of IgG anti–*B. burgdorferi* antibody are usually raised, while the level of IgM may or may not be.[13] In cases of stage 3 neurologic involvement, IgG antibodies are similarly elevated and IgM antibodies are usually normal.[16,17] Elevated serum levels of specific IgM antibody thus indicate acute infection, while elevated levels of IgG antibody may indicate either active or past infection.

Yet, neither the IFA nor the ELISA is standardized,[18,19] and both inter- and intralaboratory variability of the results of each have been reported in a number of studies.[20–22] The correct interpretation of the results of patient tests for anti–*B. burgdorferi* antibody, therefore, requires that the physician be certain of the reliability of the laboratory performing the test.

Furthermore, a positive test result may indicate only past exposure to the organism rather than active infection with it. In hyperendemic areas between 8 and 23% of residents[23-26] and 15 and 25% of those with vocational or avocational exposure[27-29] have antibodies to *B. burgdorferi* on IFA or ELISA. In several serologic surveys, moreover, it was concluded that the ratio of seropositivity from simple exposure to seropositivity from symptomatic infection is approximately 1:1, suggesting that the predictive value of a positive test result is low.[23,24] However, two more recent studies suggested that infection with *B. burgdorferi* is rarely asymptomatic, and that the majority of patients with positive serologic test results have symptoms of either early or late disease.[30,31]

Finally, false-positive reactions in both the ELISA and IFA do occur in patients with rheumatoid arthritis, Rocky Mountain spotted fever, subacute bacterial endocarditis, infectious mononucleosis, tuberculous meningitis, leptospirosis, yaws, syphilis, and both louse-borne and tick-borne relapsing fever.[6,10,11,13,27,32-34] These result most often from low titers of cross-reacting IgM antibodies. High titers of cross-reacting IgG antibodies are present only in patients with syphilis and relapsing fever.[10] Although as many as 22% of Lyme disease sera react positively in the fluorescent treponemal antibody-absorption test for syphilis,[11,35,36] and anticardiolipin antibodies can develop in patients with Lyme disease,[37] the VDRL test remains unreactive. Patients with syphilis and cross-reacting antibody, however, have positive results on reaginic tests, and relapsing fever usually can be ruled out by examining Giemsa-stained peripheral blood smears or on epidemiologic grounds.

Several modifications of the routine ELISA have been described and could increase the frequency of true-positive results, particularly in early disease, and decrease the number of false positives. These include the use of *B. burgdorferi* fractions as antigen, particularly the flagellin fraction[38-41]; the antibody capture enzyme immunoassay[42]; and preadsorption of serum with *Escherichia coli*[43] or with *Treponema reiteri*.[25,36] Although several of these methods promise increased test specificity and sensitivity, none of them is widely used at present.

Serum Immunoblots. The serum immunoblot, however, is a more sensitive and specific antibody test that is generally available.[14,32,44] A positive finding on immunoblot confirms the specificity of a positive result on ELISA or IFA. In addition, serum immunoblots are often positive earlier in both stage 1 disease[14,32,44] and stage 2 meningitis[45] than are conventional ELISAs, and the immunoblots are less often falsely positive, as long as a sufficient number of antibody bands is required for a positive result. Many normal individuals do have antibodies against *B. burgdorferi*, probably cross-reacting antibodies formed against spirochetal members of the body's normal flora. Hence, immunoblots from many normal individuals do demonstrate antibody to the 41-kd flagellin of *B. burgdorferi* or, less commonly, the 60- or 66-kd antigens,[15] as do immunoblots from some patients with rheumatic diseases, syphilis, and relapsing fever.[14] But most patients with Lyme disease have antibodies reacting with several different antigens.[44]

CSF ANTIBODY TESTS

Specific anti–*B. burgdorferi* antibody also appears in the CSF of patients with Lyme disease and neurologic abnormalities and may be detected there even when test results for serum antibody are negative.[35,46,47] Simultaneous measurement of serum and CSF antibody levels and the calculation of a CSF antibody index establish that these antibodies are synthesized intrathecally.[16,35,46–48] The most accurate method of measurement appears to be that of Hofstad et al.[49] in which serum and CSF are both diluted to the same final IgG concentration before comparing the antibody activity of the two so that the ratio is arrived at directly, eliminating the inaccuracy introduced by determining antibody titers first. But the capture ELISA on CSF may be even more accurate: It eliminates the need for diluting the two samples to the same final IgG concentration entirely since it measures the ratio of specific IgG to total IgG directly, and its absorbance value is not affected by dilution with buffer.[50,51] The capture ELISA on CSF is not in general use at present, however.

Among European patients with stage 2 neurologic abnormalities, both IgG (85%) and IgM (65%) antibodies are regularly present in CSF.[35] As many as 25% of Swedish patients with borrelial meningitis, usually those with disease of short duration ($\leq$ 3 weeks), have raised antibody titers in the CSF but not in serum, while 91% overall have CSF antibody compared with 67% with positive serum test results.[35] Among North American patients with stage 2 meningopolyneuritis, the frequency of intrathecal antibody synthesis is similar (92%), but raised IgG (46%) and IgM (38%) are less common than raised IgA (85%).[50]

Almost all patients with progressive borrelia encephalomyelitis have intrathecal synthesis of IgG anti–*B. burgdorferi* antibody, accompanied often by specific IgA antibody, and, in a few cases, in the absence of serum antibody.[16,48,50] Intrathecal antibody synthesis is less frequent (30 to 40%) among North American patients with late encephalopathy, and it is typically absent in those late cases with only peripheral nervous system abnormalities.[17,50]

Immunoblots done with CSF from patients with stage 2 meningopolyneuritis demonstrate *B. burgdorferi*–specific oligoclonal IgG in the CSF indicative of intrathecal synthesis in 80%; but, in most cases, the antibody response in the CSF is restricted to fewer proteins than in the serum.[45,52,53] The antibody response increases over time; *B. burgdorferi*–specific bands are present in 40% at 2 weeks, in 88% between 3 and 6 weeks, and in 100% after 6 weeks from onset, the number of bands increasing with disease duration.[53] The antibody bands persist at least a year after therapy despite clinical recovery. The clinical usefulness of CSF immunoblot testing is not clear however: Since there are fewer nonspecific cross-reactants in the CSF, false-positive results on CSF ELISA or IFA are rare, and there is less need for a confirmatory test.

TESTS FOR SEQUESTERED ANTIBODY

In some cases, specific serum antibody is present but sequestered in immune complexes and therefore not measurable by routine ELISA. Polyethylene glycol (PEG) precipitation of serum immune complexes, followed by dissociation in PEG-borate and analysis by specific ELISA and immunoblot, is a relatively simple technique that could improve laboratory diagnosis in seronegative patients with suspected Lyme disease.

Using this technique, Schutzer et al.[54] showed complexed anti–*B. burgdorferi* antibody in 21 (95%) of 22 seropositive patients with active Lyme disease, in all 10 seronegative patients with EM, and 4 of 12 seronegative patients with possible Lyme disease without EM. Complexed antibody was also found in seronegative patients with positive T cell–mediated immunity and in seronegative patients who later had seroconverted by follow-up. Furthermore, complexes precipitated from 5 of 5 patient samples tested contained *B. burgdorferi* antigen in addition to antibody.

The test could also improve laboratory diagnosis in patients with possible CNS Lyme disease. *B. burgdorferi*–specific immune complexes are common in the CSF of North American patients with late Lyme disease and neurologic complaints, occurring in 25 to 57% of those with cognitive impairment and fatigue.[55]

T-Cell Tests

A vigorous, specific T-cell immune response develops early in the course of Lyme disease, often before there is measurable antibody production. Once developed, it is long lasting, not related to disease activity, and unaffected by antibiotic treatment. Measurement of T-cell proliferation in response to *B. burgdorferi in vitro* can document exposure to the organism and may be useful when the results of antibody tests are inconclusive.

In one study, 14 of 17 seronegative patients with clinically active Lyme disease had a marked T-cell response to the organism.[56] A more recent report from another laboratory, however, indicated that the T-cell assay was positive in only 44% of patients with active Lyme disease, and that it was positive in addition in 4 of 9 seronegative controls who worked with *B. burgdorferi* in the laboratory.[57] Moreover, others found an unusually high frequency of reactivity in normal, unexposed individuals from endemic areas, suggesting that the test may not be specific.[58] Indeed, there is cross-reactivity with *Borrelia hermsii* and with the heat shock protein of *Mycobacterium tuberculosis*.[57]

The T-cell assay probably does have a role in the laboratory diagnosis of Lyme disease, but how great a role is not yet clear. The test is best used only when the likelihood of Lyme disease is high. The test is performed in only a few centers, however, even though it is within the capability of most modern immunology laboratories.

Clinical Diagnosis

Lyme disease should be suspected in patients with chronic lymphocytic meningitis or mild meningoencephalitis, especially when there are super-imposed cranial or peripheral neuropathies or radiculoplexopathies. Lyme disease is also likely in patients with Bell's palsy, unexplained distal axonal neuropathy, and progressive encephalomyelitis, among others. But patients with a variety of neurologic abnormalities may have nervous system Lyme disease (Table 9–1). When these abnormalities follow EM, accompany or follow Lyme arthritis or lymphocytoma, or accompany acrodermatitis chronica atrophicans (ACA), the diagnosis is usually straightforward.

Neurologic involvement in Lyme disease does occur without prior or accompanying skin or joint involvement, however. Then a number of epidemiologic clues may aid the diagnosis: a history of tick bite, travel or residence in an endemic area, and, in cases of stage 2 involvement, onset in summer.

Once it is suspected on clinical grounds, the diagnosis usually can be confirmed by demonstrating an immune response to *B. burgdorferi* in serum, CSF, or both. But no serologic measurement, regardless of titer, accurately reflects disease activity, and neither the presence of serum immunity nor the presence of T-cell reactivity to the organism is sufficient by itself to diagnose active infection. Both seropositivity and T-cell reactivity may represent only coincidental *B. burgdorferi* exposure in a patient with some other neurologic illness.

Consequently, the clinical diagnosis of definite Lyme disease involving the nervous system requires the presence of a compatible neurologic abnormality without other cause and at least one of the following: (1) a history of well-documented EM; (2) history or presence of lymphocytoma; (3) the presence of ACA; (4) serum *and* CSF reactivity, or CSF reactivity alone, against *B. burgdorferi*; (5) both other organ system involvement typical of Lyme disease and raised titers of specific serum antibody; or (6) seroconversion or fourfold rise in titer of paired serum specimens (Table 9–2). Although Lyme disease still can be suspected and antibiotic treatment prescribed if all of these criteria are not met, the diagnosis is not certain, and other possibilities should be considered.

Seronegative Lyme Disease

The detection of serum antibody against *B. burgdorferi* is the best laboratory indication of Lyme disease, but test results for serum antibodies are not always positive when neurologic abnormalities develop, especially in stage 2.[35,59] In one European series, for example, only 9 (43%) of 21 patients

Table 9–1. Neurologic Syndromes that may be Associated with Lyme Disease

Early	Late
CNS Abnormalities	
Acute aseptic meningitis	Progressive encephalomyelitis
Acute purulent meningitis*	Focal encephalitis
Chronic lymphocytic meningitis	Cerebral vasculitis
Recurrent meningitis	Stroke
Acute meningoencephalitis	Multi-infarct dementia
Acute focal encephalitis	Leukoencephalitis
Encephalomyelitis	Brain stem encephalitis
Leukoencephalitis	Hydrocephalus
Acute cerebellar ataxia	Late encephalopathy
Acute Parkinson's syndrome	Cerebellar ataxia
Hydrocephalus	Transverse myelitis
Seizure disorder	Progressive spastic para- or quadriparesis
Acute transverse myelitis	Motor neuron disease
Subacute myelitis	
Syringomyelia*	
PNS Abnormalities	
Painful radiculitis	Meningoradiculitis
Plexitis or radiculoplexitis	Radiculoplexitis
Mononeuritis simplex/multiplex	Progressive radiculoneuritis
Sensory radiculopathy	Mononeuritis simplex/multiplex
Distal symmetric polyneuritis	Distal axonopathy
Guillain-Barré syndrome	ACA-associated neuropathy
Cauda equina syndrome	Neuropathy associated with morphea
Cranial mono- or polyneuritis	and LSA†
(especially Bell's palsy)	Carpal tunnel syndrome
Ulnar nerve entrapment*	Cranial neuritis (especially nerves VII
Carpal tunnel syndrome	and VIII)
Muscle Abnormalities	
Interstitial myositis	Focal nodular myositis

*Evidence from only a few or single case reports.
†Lichen sclerosus et atrophicus.

who tested positive on CSF culture were seropositive while 9 (43%) had borderline serum antibody levels, and 3 (14%) were seronegative.[60]

In some seronegative patients with early disease, testing acute and convalescent sera may show a rise in titer,[61] but a significant change may not occur for weeks to months[62] or, rarely, years.[31] Testing paired serum can then lead to a delay in treatment if the diagnosis is not clinically certain. In others, immunoblots become positive before the ELISA or IFA[45,63]: They should be done routinely in seronegative patients when the suspicion of early nervous system Lyme disease is strong. A search for CSF antibody should be routine as well since as many as 25% of patients with borrelial meningitis may have raised titers in CSF but not in serum.[35] However, in up to 10% of patients,

Table 9–2. Diagnostic Criteria for Lyme Neuroborreliosis*

Definite Neuroborreliosis
Compatible neurologic abnormality without other cause and one or more of the following:
1. history of well-documented EM
2. history or presence of lymphocytoma
3. presence of ACA
4. serum *and* CSF immunoreactivity, or CSF reactivity alone, against *B. burgdorferi* by ELISA or immunoblot
5. both other organ system involvement typical of Lyme disease (e.g., Lyme arthritis) and serum immunoreactivity to *B. burgdorferi*
6. seroconversion or 4-fold rise in titer of antibody to *B. burgdorferi* between acute and convalescent sera

Probable Neuroborreliosis
Compatible neurologic abnormality without other cause and serum immunoreactivity to *B. burgdorferi*

Possible Neuroborreliosis
Compatible neurologic abnormality without other cause and tick bite or travel or residence in an endemic area

*Adapted from Reik L: Lyme disease, in: Scheld WM, Whitley RJ, Durack DT, eds. *Infections of the Central Nervous System*. New York: Raven Press. In press.

particularly those with disease of very short duration (1 to 3 weeks), test results for both serum and CSF antibody are negative initially,[35] and treatment will have to be prescribed on clinical grounds alone without laboratory confirmation.

Late nervous system involvement also develops in seronegative patients, though not commonly ($< 5\%$ of patients with late Lyme disease in one large clinic population).[56] Seronegative late disease occurs most commonly in patients who have received oral antibiotics early in the course, as early antibiotic treatment sometimes abrogates the antibody response to *B. burgdorferi* without eliminating it from the nervous system.[56] Seronegative patients with late disease occasionally have positive immunoblots, but not usually. In North American patients with late encephalopathy, the CSF antibody index is sometimes positive when serum antibody test results are negative,[17] while European patients with progressive encephalomyelitis rarely have CSF but not serum antibody.[64] When available, T-cell test results are positive in about 80% of seronegative patients with late disease, and can confirm exposure to the organism.[56] As in stage 2, however, some patients will have to be treated on clinical grounds alone.

Diagnosing Late Nervous System Lyme Disease

The usual dramatic neurologic manifestations of stage 2 Lyme disease generally cause no difficulty in diagnosis. But in stage 3, where the full range of nervous system abnormalities is not yet as well defined as in stage 2, the numerous and sometimes subtle neurologic disturbances can make diagnosis difficult. Nor is it certain how to best diagnose late nervous system Lyme disease once it is suspected. A positive serologic finding, while helpful, is not sufficient for diagnosis since the presence of antibody may merely indicate exposure rather than active infection, and serum antibody can persist in high titer for years after successful antibiotic therapy. While the presence of CSF antibody may be of some help, it too can persist for years after successful treatment. In addition, it is neither clear that CSF reactivity is necessary to diagnose CNS infection nor that it is the best predictor of response to treatment.

These questions are unlikely to be answered soon. Until they are, it seems prudent to test regularly for Lyme disease in patients with compatible neurologic abnormalities (see Table 9–1). In patients with a positive serum test result, the CSF should be examined and tested for antibody. Pleocytosis, elevated CSF protein, and locally synthesized anti–*B. burgdorferi* antibodies are all indications for antibiotic therapy. In patients with distal axonopathy the CSF is often normal, and treatment should be prescribed regardless. Treatment is also appropriate in seropositive patients with compatible neurologic abnormalities without other explanation and a normal CSF (probable Lyme disease), especially if the deficits are progressive. Symptoms suggesting late nervous system Lyme disease (see Table 9–1) without raised antibody titers, a history of well-documented EM, or other evidence of Lyme disease usually prove to have some other cause and typically do not respond to antibiotic treatment.

References

1. Hyde FW, Johnson RC, White TJ, Shelburne CE. Detection of antigens in urine of mice and humans infected with *Borrelia burgdorferi*, etiologic agent of Lyme disease. *J Clin Microbiol* 1989;27:58–61.
2. Feder HM Jr. Diagnostic tests for Lyme disease. *JAMA* 1990;264:693.
3. Schwan TG, Simpson WJ, Schrumpf ME, Karstens RH. Identification of *Borrelia burgdorferi* and *B. hermsii* using DNA hybridization probes. *J Clin Microbiol* 1989;27:1734–1738.
4. Rosa PA, Schwan TG. A specific and sensitive assay for the Lyme disease spirochete *Borrelia burgdorferi* using the polymerase chain reaction. *J Infect Dis* 1989;160:1018–1029.
5. Reik L, Steere AC, Bartenhagen NH, Shope RE, Malawista SE. Neurologic abnormalities of Lyme disease. *Medicine (Baltimore)* 1979;58:281–294.
6. Craft JE, Grodzicki RL, Steere AC. The antibody response in Lyme disease: Evaluation of diagnostic tests. *J Infect Dis* 1984;149:789–795.
7. Magnarelli LA, Meegan JM, Anderson JF, Chappell WA. Comparison of an indirect fluorescent-antibody test with an enzyme-linked immunosorbent assay for serological studies of Lyme disease. *J Clin Microbiol* 1984;20:181–184.
8. Magnarelli LA, Anderson JF. Early detection and persistence of antibodies to *Borrelia burgdorferi* in persons with Lyme disease. *Zentralbl Bakteriol Mikrobiol Hyg [A]* 1986;263:392–399.
9. Magnarelli LA. Serologic diagnosis of Lyme disease. *Ann NY Acad Sci* 1988;539:154–161.
10. Magnarelli LA, Anderson JF. Enzyme-linked immunosorbent assays for the detection of class-specific immunoglobulins to *Borrelia burgdorferi*. *Am J Epidemiol* 1988;127:818–825.
11. Russell H, Sampson JS, Schmid GP, Wilkinson HW, Plikaytis B. Enzyme-linked immunosorbent assay for Lyme disease. *J Infect Dis* 1984;149:465–470.

12. Cutler SJ, Wright DJM. Comparison of immunofluorescence and enzyme-linked immunosorbent assays for diagnosing Lyme disease. *J Clin Pathol* 1989;42:869–871.
13. Steere AC, Grodzicki RL, Kornblatt AN, et al. The spirochetal etiology of Lyme disease. *N Engl J Med* 1983;308:740–742.
14. Craft JE, Fischer DK, Shimamato GT, Steere AC. Antigens of *Borrelia burgdorferi* recognized during Lyme disease: Appearance of a new immunoglobulin M response and expansion of the immunoglobulin G response late in the illness. *J Clin Invest* 1986;78:934–939.
15. Dattwyler RJ, Volkman DJ, Luft BJ. Immunologic aspects of Lyme borreliosis. *Rev Infect Dis* 1989;11(suppl 6):S1494–S1498.
16. Ackermann R, Rehse-Küpper B, Gollmer E, Schmidt R. Chronic neurologic manifestations of erythema migrans borreliosis. *Ann NY Acad Sci* 1988;539:16–23.
17. Halperin JJ, Luft BJ, Anand AK, et al. Lyme neuroborreliosis: Central nervous system manifestations. *Neurology* 1989;29:753–759.
18. Wilkinson HW, Russell H, Sampson JS. Caveats on using nonstandardized serologic tests for Lyme disease. *J Clin Microbiol* 1985;21:291.
19. Magnarelli LA. Quality of Lyme disease tests. *JAMA* 1989;262:3464–3465.
20. Hedberg CW, Osterholm MT, MacDonald KL, White KE. An interlaboratory study of antibody to *Borrelia burgdorferi*. *J Infect Dis* 1987;155:1325–1327.
21. Schwartz BS, Goldstein MD, Ribeiro JMC, Schulze TL, Shahied SI. Antibody testing in Lyme disease: A comparison of results in four laboratories. *JAMA* 1989;262:3431–3434.
22. Luger SW, Krauss E. Serologic tests for Lyme disease: Interlaboratory variability. *Arch Intern Med* 1990;150:761–763.
23. Hanrahan JP, Benach JL, Coleman JL, et al. Incidence and cumulative frequency of endemic Lyme disease in a community. *J Infect Dis* 1984;150:489–496.
24. Steere AC, Taylor E, Wilson ML, Levine JF, Spielman A. Longitudinal assessment of the clinical and epidemiological features of Lyme disease in a defined population. *J Infect Dis* 1986;154:295–300.
25. Dlesk A, Broste SK, Marx JJ, McCarty PA, Mitchell PD, Motszko CS. Lyme serologies (LS) by indirect fluorescent antibody assay (IFA) and enzyme-linked immunosorbent assay (ELISA) in normal residents from an endemic area. *Arthritis Rheum* 1988;31(suppl):S98.
26. Dlesk A, Broste SK, McCarty PA, Mitchell PD. Prevalence of Lyme seropositivity by indirect immunofluorescent antibody assay (IFA) in normal adult individuals from an endemic area. *Arthritis Rheum* 1988;31(suppl):S98.
27. Wilske B, Schierz G, Preac-Mursic V, Weber K, Pfister H-W, Einhäupl K. Serological diagnosis of erythema migrans disease and related disorders. *Infection* 1984;12:331–337.
28. Münchhoff P, Wilske B, Preac-Mursic V, Schierz G. Antibodies against *Borrelia burgdorferi* in Bavarian forest workers. *Zentralbl Bakteriol Mikrobiol Hyg [A]* 1986;263:412–419.
29. Zhioua E, Gern L, Aeschlimann A. Follow-up of "Lyme-titers" and clinical associations: A prospective study on Lyme borreliosis. *Arthritis Rheum* 1988;31(suppl):S98.
30. Lipschitz R, Gardella JE, Gorevic D, Dattwyler RJ. Serological and clinical evidence of occult Lyme borreliosis. *Arthritis Rheum* 1988;31(suppl):S97.
31. Lastavica CC, Wilson ML, Berardi VP, Spielman A, Deblinger RD. Rapid emergence of a focal epidemic of Lyme disease in coastal Massachusetts. *N Engl J Med* 1989;320:133–137.
32. Barbour AG, Burgdorfer W, Grunwalt E, Steere AC. Antibodies of patients with Lyme disease to components of the *Ixodes dammini* spirochete. *J Clin Invest* 1983;72:504–515.
33. Magnarelli LA, Anderson JF, Johnson RC. Cross-reactivity in serological tests for Lyme disease and other spirochetal infections. *J Infect Dis* 1987;156:183–188.
34. Kaell A, Volkman D, Gorevic P, Bennett R, Hamburger M, Dattwyler R. Positive Lyme serology in subacute bacterial endocarditis: a study of four patients. *JAMA* 1990;264:2916–2918.
35. Stiernstedt GT, Granström M, Hederstedt B, Sköldenberg B. Diagnosis of spirochetal meningitis by enzyme-linked immunosorbent assay and indirect immunofluorescent assay in serum and cerebrospinal fluid. *J Clin Microbiol* 1985;21:819–825.
36. Hunter EF, Russell H, Farshy CE, Sampson JS, Larsen SA. Evaluation of sera from patients with Lyme disease in the fluorescent treponemal antibody-absorption test for syphilis. *Sex Transm Dis* 1986;13:232–236.
37. Mackworth-Young CG, Harris EN, Steere AC, et al. Anticardiolipin antibodies in Lyme disease. *Arthritis Rheum* 1988;31:1052–1056.
38. Magnarelli LA, Anderson JF, Barbour AG. Enzyme-linked immunosorbent assays for Lyme disease: Reactivity of subunits of *Borrelia burgdorferi*. *J Infect Dis* 1989;159:43–49.
39. Coleman JL, Benach JL. Isolation of antigenic components from the Lyme disease spirochete: Their role in early diagnosis. *J Infect Dis* 1987;155:756–765.

40. Hansen K, Hindersson P, Pederson NS. Measurement of antibodies to the *Borrelia burgdorferi* flagellum improves serodiagnosis in Lyme disease. *J Clin Microbiol* 1988;26:338–346.
41. Hansen K, Åsbrink E. Serodiagnosis of erythema migrans and acrodermatitis chronica atrophicans by the *Borrelia burgdorferi* flagellum enzyme-linked immunosorbent assay. *J Clin Microbiol* 1989;27:545–551.
42. Berardi VP, Weeks KE, Steere AC. Serodiagnosis of early Lyme disease: Analysis of IgM and IgG antibody responses by using an antibody-capture enzyme immunoassay. *J Infect Dis* 1988;158:754–760.
43. Fawcett PT, O'Brien AE, Doughty RA. An adsorption procedure to increase the specificity of enzyme-linked immunosorbent assays for Lyme disease without decreasing sensitivity. *Arthritis Rheum* 1989;32:1041–1044.
44. Grodzicki RL, Steere AC. Comparison of immunoblotting and indirect enzyme-linked immunosorbent assay using different antigen preparations for diagnosing early Lyme disease. *J Infect Dis* 1988;157:790–797.
45. Karlsson M, Möllegård I, Stiernstedt G, Henriksson AM, Wretlind B. Characterization of antibody response in patients with *Borrelia* meningitis. *Serodiagn Immunother Infect Dis* 1988;2:375–386.
46. Murray N, Kristoferitsch W, Stanek G, Steck AJ. Specificity of CSF antibodies against components of *Borrelia burgdorferi* in patients with meningopolyneuritis Garin-Bujadoux-Bannwarth. *J Neurol* 1986;233:224–227.
47. Wilske B, Schierz G, Preac-Mursic V, et al. Intrathecal production of specific antibodies against *Borrelia burgdorferi* in patients with lymphocytic meningoradiculitis (Bannwarth's syndrome). *J Infect Dis* 1986;153:304–314.
48. Rehse-Küpper B, Ackerman R. Demonstration of locally synthesized *Borrelia* antibodies in cerebrospinal fluid. *Zentralbl Bakteriol Mikrobiol Hyg [A]* 1986;263:407–411.
49. Hofstad H, Matre R, Nyland H, Ulvestad E. Bannwarth's syndrome: Serum and CSF IgG antibodies against *Borrelia burgdorferi* examined by ELISA. *Acta Neurol Scand* 1987;75:37–45.
50. Steere AC, Berardi VP, Weeks KE, Logigian EL, Ackermann R. Evaluation of the intrathecal antibody response to *Borrelia burgdorferi* as a diagnostic test for Lyme neuroborreliosis. *J Infect Dis* 1990;161:1203–1209.
51. von Stedingk L-V, von Stedingk M, Brauner A, et al. Intrathecally produced antibodies to *Borrelia burgdorferi* measured by IgG capture ELISA. Presented at the Fourth International Conference on Lyme Disease; June 18–21, 1990; Stockholm, Sweden.
52. Martin R, Martens U, Sticht-Groh V, Dörries R, Krüger H. Persistent intrathecal secretion of oligoclonal, *Borrelia burgdorferi*-specific IgG in chronic meningoradiculomyelitis. *J Neurol* 1988;235:229–233.
53. Hansen K, Cruz M, Link H. Oligoclonal *Borrelia burgdorferi*-specific IgG antibodies in cerebrospinal fluid in Lyme neuroborreliosis. *J Infect Dis* 1990;161:1194–1202.
54. Schutzer SE, Coyle PK, Belman AL, Golightly MG, Drulle J. Sequestration of antibody to *Borrelia burgdorferi* in immune complexes in seronegative Lyme disease. *Lancet* 1990;1:312–315.
55. Coyle PK, Krupp LB, Belman AL. Immune correlates of cognitive impairment in Lyme disease. *Neurology* 1990;40(suppl 1):332.
56. Dattwyler RJ, Volkman DJ, Luft BJ, Halperin JJ, Thomas J, Golightly MG. Seronegative Lyme disease: Dissociation of specific T- and B-lymphocyte responses to *Borrelia burgdorferi*. *N Engl J Med* 1988;319:1441–1446.
57. Dressler F, Yoshinari NH, Steere AC. Evaluation of the T-cell proliferative assay as a diagnostic test in Lyme disease. Presented at the Fourth International Conference on Lyme Borreliosis; June 18–21, 1990; Stockholm, Sweden.
58. Zoschke D, Kolstoe J, Skemp A. Positive lymphocyte proliferation to *Borrelia* in Lyme disease—a cautionary note. *Arthritis Rheum* 1989;32:S46.
59. Stiernstedt G. Tick-borne borrelia infection in Sweden. *Scand J Infect Dis Suppl* 1975;45:1–70.
60. Preac-Mursic V. Presented at the Fourth International Conference on Lyme Borreliosis; June 18–21, 1990; Stockholm, Sweden.
61. Feder HM, Zalneraitis EL, Reik L. Lyme disease: Acute focal meningoencephalitis in a child. *Pediatrics* 1988;82:931–934.
62. Magnarelli LA. Laboratory diagnosis of Lyme disease. *Rheum Dis Clin North Am* 1989;15:735–745.
63. Guy EC, Turner AM. Seronegative neuroborreliosis. *Lancet* 1989;1:441.
64. Ackermann R. Tertiary neuroborreliosis: The enlarging spectrum. Presented at the Fourth International Conference on Lyme Borreliosis; June 18–21, 1990; Stockholm, Sweden.

10

Treatment

The goal of antibiotic therapy in Lyme disease is to eradicate *Borrelia burgdorferi* and thereby cure erythema migrans (EM) and its associated symptoms; prevent the development of late skin, joint, heart, and nervous system disease; and eliminate these late complications when they do occur. But the best antibiotic regimens for doing so are not certain.

Treatment of Early Localized Disease

Antibiotics were used successfully to treat Lyme disease first in the 1950s when Hollström[1,2] and Hellerström[3] prescribed penicillin for European patients with EM and lymphocytic meningitis. Early trials in the United States, undertaken before the cause of Lyme disease became known, also demonstrated a benefit from antibiotic treatment.[4,5] EM resolved sooner (2 to 4 days compared to 10 days) in patients treated with oral penicillin or tetracycline than in untreated patients or those treated with erythromycin, and treatment with each of these antibiotics, including erythromycin, significantly reduced the incidence of late complications, tetracycline being most effective.

Several subsequent reports from Europe described similar success in treating EM with these oral antibiotics.[6,7] But several others suggested that a substantial number of patients with early disease, particularly those with more severe initial illness, may not be cured by oral therapy.[8–10] Many treated patients continued to have symptoms (recurrent headaches, arthralgias, musculoskeletal pain, and lethargy), sometimes recurring over several years, and some developed late extracutaneous complications, including nervous system disease.[11] Confirming this suspicion, *B. burgdorferi* has now been isolated from skin biopsy specimens taken as long as 3 months after the end of therapy from patients treated with oral antibiotics for EM,[12] and from joint fluid obtained 2 months after oral treatment of facial palsy.[13]

Tests of *in vitro* antibiotic sensitivity promise to improve the treatment of Lyme disease, however. Tests in several laboratories have now shown that *B. burgdorferi* is sensitive to a variety of antibiotics,[14–20] although only a limited number of strains have been tested so far, and testing methods have not been standardized.[21,22] The spirochete is most sensitive *in vitro* to ceftriaxone, cefotaxime, erythromycin, and several newer investigational macrolide antibiotics—azithromycin, clarithromycin, josamycin, and roxithromycin. It is also sensitive, though less so, to tetracycline, minocycline, doxycycline, amoxicillin alone or with clavulanate, mezlocillin, imipenem, lincomycin, chloramphenicol, and ciprofloxacin. It is only moderately sensitive to penicillin, however, and is resistant to ofloxacin, gentamicin, amikacin, and trimethoprim.

B. *burgdorferi* antibiotic sensitivities measured *in vivo* in experimentally infected laboratory animals generally parallel those measured *in vitro*.[16,17,20] Ceftriaxone, cefotaxime, and the tetracyclines are most active, while penicillin remains only moderately so (although more recent experiments using more frequent antibiotic administration have shown penicillin to be highly effective in infected gerbils[23]). Azithromycin and roxithromycin also remain effective in animal models,[20,24] but erythromycin is much less active *in vivo* than it is *in vitro*.[16,17]

Moreover, data from these tests suggest that oral therapy of early disease may have failed in some cases because penicillin and tetracycline are not the best antibiotics to treat it. The minimal inhibitory concentrations of both antibiotics for some strains of *B. burgdorferi* are equal to or above the serum concentration achieved by oral administration.[25]

Sensitivity data also suggest that amoxicillin and doxycycline are better choices for early oral therapy. Amoxicillin is more active against *B. burgdorferi* than penicillin V and more reliably absorbed than penicillin G,[26] and it can achieve effective levels in the CSF when given orally with probenecid.[27] Similarly, doxycycline achieves higher tissue levels than tetracycline, particularly in the brain where it reaches concentrations five times those of equivalent doses of tetracycline; it has fewer gastrointestinal side effects; and, because of its longer half-life, it can be given on a twice daily schedule.[27–29]

More recent clinical trials have focused on these and other alternatives to penicillin and tetracycline, therefore. Both oral doxycycline (100 mg), twice daily for 21 days, and oral amoxicillin (500 mg) plus probenecid (500 mg), three times daily for 21 days, have been shown to cure 85% of patients with EM, with the remainder having arthralgias (7%), fatigue (4%), or both (4%) when evaluated 3 months after treatment.[30] Again, late complaints are most common (29%) among patients presenting with more severe disease— multiple EM or EM with fever and constitutional symptoms. Among the newer macrolide antibiotics, josamycin is effective in treating EM,[31] while roxithromycin is not.[32] Another new approach, investigated by Weber et al.[33] is the treatment of more severe early disease with intramuscular ceftriaxone

(1 g daily for 5 days). Ceftriaxone appears to be superior to oral penicillin in these cases but not in those of milder disease.

Although there clearly are some uncertainties about the optimum treatment for early disease, it is also clear that antibiotic treatment of early disease is the best way to prevent later nervous system involvement. Currently, the best choices for the treatment of early disease appear to be doxycycline for adults, with amoxicillin as an alternative, and amoxicillin in children (Table 10–1). There is no good alternative to amoxicillin in children with penicillin allergy, but erythromycin is usually prescribed. In the future, other macrolides may substitute for it. No matter which antibiotic is chosen, treatment should be prescribed for a minimum of 10 days, but longer treatment (up to 30 days) may be required if the initial symptoms are more severe or relapse occurs after the cessation of treatment, as sometimes occurs. Approximately 15% of patients treated in this way develop an intensification of symptoms during the first 24 hours of therapy (Jarisch-Herxheimer reaction),[5] but this requires no special treatment other than general supportive measures.

Treatment of Nervous System Disease

Neurologic Abnormalities of Early Lyme Disease

Once neurologic abnormalities develop, parenteral antibiotic therapy is normally required (see Table 10–1). In stage 2, intravenous penicillin therapy is usually successful, and it has been used extensively[34–38] since Steere et al.[39] reported the treatment with high-dose intravenous aqueous penicillin G (20 million units daily for 10 days) of 12 patients with meningitis, all of whom improved within 7 to 10 days.

A few patients with stage 2 neurologic disease have failed to improve with intravenous penicillin therapy, however, responding instead to intravenous cefotaxime (2 g three times daily for 10 days),[40] ceftriaxone (2 g once or twice a day for 14 days),[41] or chloramphenicol (1 g four times daily for 10 days).[42] But in a randomized trial, cefotaxime was no more effective than penicillin G in 21 patients with stage 2 meningopolyneuritis[43]; in one additional trial involving 33 patients, the effectiveness of cefotaxime and ceftriaxone was also equal.[44]

Intravenous doxycycline (200 mg on day 1, then 100 mg daily for 10 days) also has been used to treat stage 2 neurologic disease,[36] and it has been found to be as effective as intravenous penicillin in a controlled trial involving 75 patients.[45] Since equivalent blood and CSF levels are achieved when doxycycline is given either orally or intravenously,[46] oral doxycycline therapy should be effective as well. Indeed, in one small study, oral doxycycline therapy (100 mg twice daily for 10 to 20 days) was curative in eight patients with stage 2 meningopolyneuritis.[47] In one other,[48] however, doxycycline concentrations in CSF exceeded the estimated mean inhibitory concentration

Table 10–1.   Antibiotic Therapy of Lyme Disease:
Treatment of Early Disease and Neurologic Abnormalities

Manifestation	Treatment
Early infection	
Localized (stage 1)	
Adults	Doxycycline, 100 mg po BID × 10–30 d*
	Amoxicillin, 500 mg po QID × 10– 30d†
Children (≤ 8 yrs)	Amoxicillin, 30–40 mg/kg/d in 4 divided doses × 10–30 d
	Erythromycin, 30 mg/kg/d in 4 divided doses × 10–30 d for patients with penicillin allergy
Disseminated (stage 2)	
Bell's palsy	Oral antibiotics as for stage 1
Other neurologic involvement	
Adults	Penicillin G, 20–24 million units/d iv × 10–14 d
	Ceftriaxone, 2 g/d iv × 2–4 wk
	Cefotaxime, 2 g iv TID × 2–4 wk
	Doxycycline, 100–200 mg po BID × 10–30 d
Children	Penicillin G, 250,000 units/kg/d iv in divided doses q4h × 10–14 d
	Ceftriaxone, 50–80 mg/kg/d iv × 2–4 wk
Late infection (stage 3)	
Progressive encephalomyelitis, late encephalopathy, or polyneuropathy	
Adults	iv Penicillin, ceftriaxone, or cefotaxime as for stage 2
	Doxycycline, 100–200 mg po BID for 30 d
Children	iv Penicillin or ceftrixone as for stage 2

*The duration of treatment with this and other regimens depends on clinical response.
†May be combined with probenecid, 500 mg po QID.

for *B. burgdorferi* in 90% of patients treated with 200 mg twice daily but in only 25% of patients treated with 100 mg twice daily, suggesting that treatment with the higher dose may be preferable in patients with nervous system disease.

Still, most patients with stage 2 neurologic disease will respond to high-dose intravenous penicillin G, especially if the meninges are inflamed. When patients with meningopolyneuritis are treated parenterally, pain and fever may worsen temporarily in the first 18 to 24 hours,[39] but severe Herxheimer reactions have not been described. Once treatment has begun, meningismus, systemic symptoms, and radicular pain all begin to improve within days, but some patients continue to have arthralgias, musculoskeletal pain, and fatigue.[38,39,43,45] Motor deficits resolve more slowly (mean recovery time, 8 weeks) and sometimes incompletely. CNS abnormalities are arrested by treatment and may improve slowly, but some residual deficit is common in severe cases.[35,38,39] CSF abnormalities are usually less marked by the end of treatment, but normalization of the cell count can take months and the protein a year or more.[38,39,43] Specific antibody can persist in CSF for at least 6 months.[43,45]

Failure of meningeal symptoms to improve by the end of 2 weeks of treatment or of CSF pleocytosis to diminish should prompt longer treatment or a change of antibiotic. In some cases, 10 days to 2 weeks of therapy is insufficient. *B. burgdorferi* was isolated from the CSF of one patient 7 months after 10 days of ceftriaxone therapy for meningopolyneuritis, and from the CSF of two others treated with high-dose intravenous penicillin for 10 to 14 days at 3 and 7 months after therapy.[12] One additional patient developed iridocyclitis and meningoencephalitis 4 months after 10 days of treatment with intravenous ceftriaxone for Lyme arthritis.[49]

Not every patient with stage 2 neurologic disease needs parenteral antibiotic therapy, though. Facial palsy can be treated adequately with oral antibiotics when it occurs without meningeal inflammation.[39,50] If there is no pleocytosis, CSF protein abnormality, or intrathecal antibody synthesis, oral doxycycline or amoxicillin can be prescribed as for stage 1 disease.

Neurologic Abnormalities of Late Lyme Disease

Like stage 2 meningopolyneuritis, progressive borrelia encephalomyelitis responds to high-dose intravenous penicillin[36,51] or intravenous doxycycline[45] with resolution of pleocytosis and reduction of CSF protein content within 3 months, but specific antibody can persist in the CSF for a year or more. The clinical signs in most patients are stabilized by treatment or regress partially: Only a few patients become clinically normal.

The response to intravenous penicillin is less consistent in patients with other stage 3 neurologic abnormalities. Treatment with intravenous ceftriaxone is more effective. In a randomized trial, Dattwyler et al. compared intravenous treatment with either penicillin or ceftriaxone in 23 patients with arthritis, peripheral neuropathy, and/or encephalopathy.[52] Five of 10 penicillin-treated patients, but only 1 of 13 ceftriaxone-treated patients, failed to improve; 3 of 4 penicillin failures later responded to ceftriaxone.

In a subsequent open trial, moreover, 27 of 31 patients with similar late disease responded to ceftriaxone.[52] Those who failed to respond were slightly older, had had the illness slightly longer, and were more likely to have received earlier steroid therapy.

Recovery after ceftriaxone therapy in late disease is slow, however.[52–54] In patients with neuropathy, resolution of electrophysiologic abnormalities and clinical signs and symptoms can take 6 months, although some improvement may be evident 2 months after treatment. The time to recovery of cerebral symptoms and neuropsychologic test abnormalities is similar: Little change is apparent during the course of treatment itself.

The best treatment for the neuropathy associated with acrodermatitis chronica atrophicans (ACA) is not known, but comparison with the distal axonopathy of North American late Lyme disease suggests that intravenous ceftriaxone should be effective.

Indeed, ceftriaxone (2 g daily for 2 weeks) appears to be the drug of choice in patients with stage 3 neurologic involvement at present (see Table 10–1). While penicillin is adequate in many patients, particularly those with progressive borrelia encephalomyelitis, it isn't always. Furthermore, the long half-life of ceftriaxone permits once daily dosing, thus allowing outpatient treatment. Most penicillin-allergic patients can still receive ceftriaxone, but the first dose probably should be administered in the hospital or physician's office in case a life-threatening reaction does occur. If allergy to ceftriaxone does develop, oral doxycycline (100 to 200 mg twice daily for 4 weeks) can be prescribed. In either case, if there is no response to treatment, or relapse occurs after an initial good response, retreatment for a longer period of time should be considered.

The use of corticosteroids in addition to antibiotics to treat nervous system Lyme disease is not recommended. While early studies did suggest that steroid therapy could promptly resolve radicular pain in meningopoly-neuritis, one small double-blind study found that the pain of men-ingopolyneuritis resolved almost as quickly with antibiotic therapy alone.[55] Since there is concern that prior steroid treatment may interfere with the response to antibiotics in late disease,[52] it seems prudent not to prescribe corticosteroids for Lyme disease at present.

References

1. Hollström E. Successful treatment of erythema chronicum migrans Afzelius. *Acta Derm Venereol (Stockh)* 1951;31:235–243.
2. Hollström E. Penicillin treatment of erythema chronicum migrans Afzelius. *Acta Derm Venereol (Stockh)* 1958;38:285–289.
3. Hellerström S. Erythema chronicum migrans Afzelius with meningitis. *Acta Derm Venereol (Stockh)* 1951;31:227–234.
4. Steere AC, Malawista SE, Newman JH, Spieler PN, Bartenhagen NH. Antibiotic therapy in Lyme disease. *Ann Intern Med* 1980;93:1–8.
5. Steere AC, Hutchinson GJ, Rahn DW, et al. Treatment of the early manifestations of Lyme disease. *Ann Intern Med* 1983;99:22–26.
6. Åsbrink E, Olsson I, Hovmark A. Erythema chronicum migrans Afzelius in Sweden: A study on 231 patients. *Zentralbl Bakteriol Mikrobiol Hyg [A]* 1986;263:229–236.
7. Neumann R, Aberer E, Stanek G. Treatment and course of erythema chronicum migrans. *Zentralbl Bakteriol Mikrobiol Hyg [A]* 1986;263:372–376.
8. Steere AC, Green J, Hutchinson GJ, et al. Treatment of Lyme disease. *Zentralbl Bakteriol Mikrobiol Hyg [A]* 1986;263:352–356.
9. Weber K, Preac-Mursic V, Neubert U, et al. Antibiotic therapy of early European Lyme borreliosis and acrodermatitis chronica atrophicans. *Ann NY Acad Sci* 1988;539:324–325.
10. Berger BW. Treatment of erythema chronicum migrans of Lyme disease. *Ann NY Acad Sci* 1988;539:346–351.
11. Dattwyler RJ, Halperin JJ. Failure of tetracycline therapy in early Lyme disease. *Arthritis Rheum* 1987;30:448–450.

12. Preac-Mursic V, Weber K, Pfister HW, et al. Survival of *Borrelia burgdorferi* in antibiotically treated patients with Lyme borreliosis. *Infection* 1989;17:355–359.
13. Schmidli J, Hunziker T, Moesli P, Schaad UB. Cultivation of *Borrelia burgdorferi* from joint fluid three months after treatment of facial palsy due to Lyme borreliosis. *J Infect Dis* 1988;158:905–906.
14. Johnson SE, Klein GC, Schmid GP, Feeley JC. Susceptibility of the Lyme disease spirochete to seven antimicrobial agents. *Yale J Biol Med* 1984;57:549–553.
15. Berger BW, Kaplan MH, Rothenberg IR, Barbour AG. Isolation and characterization of the Lyme disease spirochete from the skin of patients with erythema chronicum migrans. *J Am Acad Dermatol* 1985;13:444–449.
16. Johnson RC, Kodner C, Russell M. *In vitro* and *in vivo* susceptibility of the Lyme disease spirochete, *Borrelia burgdorferi*, to four antimicrobial agents. *Antimicrob Agents Chemother* 1987;31:164–167.
17. Mursic VP, Wilske B, Schierz G, Holmburger M, Süss E. *In vitro* and *in vivo* susceptibility of *Borrelia burgdorferi*. *Eur J Clin Microbiol* 1987;6:424–426.
18. Preac-Mursic V, Wilske B, Schierz G, Süss E, Gross B. Comparative antimicrobial activity of the new macrolides against *Borrelia burgdorferi*. *Eur J Clin Microbiol Infect Dis* 1989;8:651–653.
19. Sambri V, Cevenini R, Massaria F, La Placa M. *In vitro* activity of antimicrobials against *Borrelia burgdorferi* and *Borrelia hermsii*. Presented at the Fourth International Conference on Lyme Borreliosis; June 18–21, 1990; Stockholm, Sweden.
20. Preac-Mursic V, Wilske B. Comparison of *in vitro* and *in vivo* activity of various antibiotics against *Borrelia burgdorferi*. Presented at the Fourth International Conference on Lyme Borreliosis; June 18–21, 1990; Stockholm, Sweden.
21. Johnson RC. Isolation techniques for spirochetes and their sensitivity to antibiotics *in vitro* and *in vivo*. *Rev Infect Dis* 1989;11(suppl 6):S1505–S1510.
22. Luft BJ, Gorevic PD, Halperin JJ, Volkman DJ, Dattwyler RJ. A perspective on the treatment of Lyme borreliosis. *Rev Infect Dis* 1989;11(suppl 6):S1518–S1525.
23. Hansen K, Lebech K, Bertelsen T, Lebech A-M. Is *Borrelia burgdorferi* a penicillin-sensitive organism? An *in vitro* and *in vivo* animal study. Presented at the Fourth International Conference on Lyme Borreliosis; June 18–21, 1990; Stockholm, Sweden.
24. Lebech A-M, Lebech K, Bertelsen T, Hansen K. Susceptibility of *Borrelia burgdorferi* to roxithromycin: An *in vitro* and *in vivo* animal study. Presented at the Fourth International Conference on Lyme Borreliosis; June 18–21, 1990; Stockholm, Sweden.
25. Luft BJ, Volkman DJ, Halperin JJ, Dattwyler RJ. New chemotherapeutic approaches in the treatment of Lyme borreliosis. *Ann NY Acad Sci* 1988;539:352–361.
26. Neu HC. A perspective on therapy of Lyme infection. *Ann NY Acad Sci* 1988;539:314–316.
27. Faber WR, Bos JD, Rietra TJ, Fass J, van Eljk VW. Treponemicidal levels of amoxicillin in cerebrospinal fluid after oral administration. *Sex Transm Dis* 1983;10:148–150.
28. Barza M, Brown RB, Shanks C, Gamble C, Weinstein L. Relation between lipophilicity and pharmacological behavior of minocycline, doxycycline, tetracycline, and oxytetracycline in dogs. *Antimicrob Agents Chemother* 1975;8:713–720.
29. Yim CW, Flynn NM, Fitzgerald FT. Penetration of oral doxycycline into the cerebrospinal fluid of patients with latent or neurosyphilis. *Antimicrob Agents Chemother* 1985;28:347–348.
30. Dattwyler R, Volkman D, Platkin S, Conaty S, Luft B. Amoxicillin plus probenecid compared to doxycycline for the treatment of erythema migrans (EM). Presented at the Fourth International Conference on Lyme Borreliosis; June 18–21, 1990; Stockholm, Sweden.
31. Trevisan G, Cinco M. *In vitro* and *in vivo* activity of josamycin against *Borrelia burgdorferi*. Presented at the Fourth International Conference on Lyme Borreliosis; June 18–21, 1990; Stockholm, Sweden.
32. Hovmark A, Olsson I, Åsbrink E, Olsson E, Halkier-Sörensen L, Hansen K. A comparative study of the efficacy of roxithromycin and phenoxymethylpenicillin in the treatment of erythema migrans. Presented at the Fourth International Conference on Lyme Borreliosis; June 18–21, 1990; Stockholm, Sweden.
33. Weber K, Preac-Mursic V, Wilske B, Thurmayr R, Neubert U, Scherwitz C. Randomized comparison between ceftriaxone and oral penicillin for the treatment of erythema migrans. Presented at the Fourth International Conference on Lyme Borreliosis; June 18–21, 1990; Stockholm, Sweden.
34. Sköldenberg B, Stiernstedt G, Garde A, Kolmodin G, Carlström A, Nord CE. Chronic meningitis caused by a penicillin-sensitive microorganism? *Lancet* 1983;2:75–78.

35. Stiernstedt GT, Sköldenberg BR, Vandvik B, et al. Chronic meningitis and Lyme disease in Sweden. *Yale J Biol Med* 1984;57:491–497.
36. Kohlhepp W, Mertens H-G, Oschmann P. Acute and chronic illness after tick-bite *Borrelia burgdorferi* infections: Results of treatment. *Zentralbl Bakteriol Mikrobiol Hyg [A]* 1986;263: 365–371.
37. Kristoferitsch W, Baumhackl V, Sluga E, Stanek G, Zeiler K. High-dose penicillin therapy in meningopolyneuritis Garin-Bujadoux-Bannwarth: Clinical and cerebrospinal fluid data. *Zentralbl Bakteriol Mikrobiol Hyg [A]* 1986;263:357–364.
38. Sköldenberg B, Stiernstedt G, Karlsson M, Wretlind B, Svenungsson B. Treatment of Lyme borreliosis with emphasis on neurological disease. *Ann NY Acad Sci* 1988;539:317–323.
39. Steere AC, Pachner AR, Malawista SE. Neurologic abnormalities of Lyme disease: Successful treatment with high-dose intravenous penicillin. *Ann Intern Med* 1983;99:767–772.
40. Pal GS, Baker JT, Wright DJM. Penicillin-resistant *Borrelia* encephalitis responding to cefo-taxime. *Lancet* 1988;1:50–51.
41. Dattwyler RJ, Halperin JJ, Pass H, Luft BJ. Ceftriaxone as effective therapy in refractory Lyme disease. *J Infect Dis* 1987;155:1322–1325.
42. Diringer MN, Halperin JJ, Dattwyler RJ. Lyme meningoencephalitis—report of a severe, penicillin-resistant case. *Arthritis Rheum* 1987;30:705–708.
43. Pfister H-W, Preac-Mursic V, Wilske B, Einhäupl M. Cefotaxime vs penicillin G for acute neurologic manifestations in Lyme borreliosis: A prospective randomized study. *Arch Neurol* 1989;46:1190–1194.
44. Pfister H-W, Preac-Mursic V, Wilske B, Einhäupl KM, Schielke E, Sörgel F. Randomized comparison of ceftriaxone and cefotaxime in Lyme neuroborreliosis. Presented at the Fourth International Conference on Lyme Borreliosis; June 18–21, 1990; Stockholm, Sweden.
45. Kohlhepp W, Oschmann P, Mertens H-G. Treatment of Lyme borreliosis: Randomized comparison of doxycycline and penicillin G. *J Neurol* 1989;236:464–469.
46. Leibowitz BJ, Hakes JL, Cahn MM, Levy EJ. Doxycycline blood levels in normal subjects after intravenous and oral administration. *Curr Ther Res* 1972;14:820–832.
47. Dovetall L, Alestig K, Hanner P, Norkrans G, Hagberg L. The use of doxycycline in nervous system *Borrelia burgdorferi* infection. *Scand J Infect Dis Suppl* 1988;53:74–79.
48. Dovetall L, Hagberg L. Penetration of doxycycline into cerebrospinal fluid in patients treated for suspected Lyme neuroborreliosis. *Antimicrob Agents Chemother* 1989;33:1078–1080.
49. Valesová M, Trnavsky K, Alusik S, Janousek J, Hulinská D, Jirous J. Ceftriaxone in the treatment of Lyme arthritis. Presented at the Fourth International Conference on Lyme Borreliosis; June 18–21, 1990; Stockholm, Sweden.
50. Steere AC. Lyme disease. *N Engl J Med* 1989;321:586–596.
51. Ackermann R, Rehse-Küpper B, Gollmer E, Schmidt R. Chronic neurologic manifestations of erythema migrans borreliosis. *Ann NY Acad Sci* 1988;539:16–23.
52. Dattwyler RJ, Halperin JJ, Volkman DJ, Luft BJ. Treatment of late Lyme borreliosis—randomized comparison of ceftriaxone and penicillin. *Lancet* 1988;1:1191–1194.
53. Halperin JJ, Little BW, Coyle PK, Dattwyler RJ. Lyme disease: Cause of a treatable peripheral neuropathy. *Neurology* 1987;37:1700–1706.
54. Halperin JJ, Pass HL, Anand AK, Luft BJ, Volkman DJ, Dattwyler RJ. Nervous system abnormalities in Lyme disease. *Ann NY Acad Sci* 1988;539:24–34.
55. Pfister HW, Einhäupl KM, Franz P, Garner C. Corticosteroids for radicular pain in Bann-warth's syndrome: A double-blind, randomized, placebo-controlled trial. *Ann NY Acad Sci* 1988;539:485–487.

11

Prevention

The best chance for reducing the burden of neurologic illness due to Lyme disease lies in the prevention of infection. While vaccination of those at risk is potentially the best way to do so, no vaccine is available for human use, although Syrian hamsters[1] and laboratory mice[2] have been successfully immunized against *Borrelia burgdorferi*, and a commercial vaccine has been approved for use in dogs. Consequently, prevention of the disease in humans depends at present on reducing the incidence of infective tick bites. The methods for doing so include personal protection and the reduction of tick populations through biologic or chemical control, environmental modification and physical control, and control of their vertebrate hosts.

Personal Protection

The best way to prevent Lyme disease is to avoid tick-infested areas during the warmer late spring and early summer months when the nymphs are most active.[3-5] Heavy infestation with *Ixodes dammini*, the most important North American vector, is most likely in woodlands, shrub, and areas of transitional vegetation on the edges of woods and fields, especially along trails in areas used extensively by deer.[3-6] Visiting these areas is less likely to be a problem at other times of the year. During fall and winter, when the adults are active, more protective clothing is likely to be worn, and the adults are larger, more easily noticed, and less common than the nymphs. The larvae, which feed in late summer, are not infected and pose no risk.

In North America, however, infected ticks are often common in suburbs near large tracts of undeveloped woodlands.[7] In one such area, Westchester County, New York, nearly 70% of reported tick bites actually occur in the bitten individuals' own yards.[8] Some degree of exposure is inevitable, therefore, even if other high-risk areas are avoided.

If exposure is inevitable, other personal protective measures can help.[4,5] Nymphs of *I. dammini* are typically located at ground level, often in leaf litter, while adults are usually at knee level in the forest understory. Both most often gain access to human hosts by climbing up the legs. Wearing long pants with the cuffs tightly taped or tucked into socks reduces the risk of being bitten. A tucked-in, long-sleeved shirt with snug-fitting collar and cuffs is also advisable, as is a hat. Smooth close-weave fabrics are harder for the ticks to crawl on than coarser open-weave fabrics, and light colors make spotting the ticks easier. Sitting or lying on the ground should be avoided.

Repellents can provide additional protection. The most widely available of these, *N,N*-diethyl-m-toluamide or deet, repels ticks when impregnated into clothing.[4,5,9,10] In one study, a 1-minute application of 20% and 30% deet to military uniforms provided 86% and 92% protection against *I. dammini* in an area of Cape Cod, Massachusetts, heavily infested with the tick.[10] Deet also repels ticks when applied to the skin, but it loses its effect within 1 to several hours due to absorption, evaporation, rain, sweating, or wiping, and it must be reapplied to maintain effectiveness.[9] Moreover, deet is not entirely benign. It has been associated with local bullous eruptions and contact urticaria at the site of application.[9] In addition, it is absorbed through the skin into the systemic circulation (10 to 15% of each dose can be recovered from the urine), and anaphylaxis, toxic encephalopathy, and grand mal seizures have occurred when deet has been applied at higher concentrations or after its excessive or prolonged use.[9]

A new acaricide, permethrin, kills ticks on contact and provides high levels of protection against *I. dammini* when it is applied to clothing.[9,10] The same study that assayed the effect of deet against *I. dammini* showed that a 1-minute application of 0.5% permethrin to clothing provided 100% protection against the tick.[10] It also appears to be safer than deet. It is poorly absorbed and then rapidly inactivated by ester hydrolysis, skin toxicity has been uncommon, and adverse systemic effects have not been reported.[9] The best defense against tick bites thus seems to be the use of protective clothing treated with permethrin plus the judicious use of deet in low concentrations on exposed skin.

Several additional protective measures may help.[4,5] Clothing should be brushed off before entering the house after outdoor activity, and the clothes should be removed immediately and washed. Exposed individuals should shower promptly after coming inside, and adults should inspect their children and themselves for ticks, especially in hair-covered areas, around hairlines, in the ears, around the eyes, under arms, in body folds, and behind the knees.

If a tick is found and attachment has occurred, disease transmission can still be prevented: Transmission is rare after fewer than 24 hours of attachment.[11] The tick should be removed as soon as possible by grasping it with fine tweezers as close to the skin as possible and pulling gently.[4,5] Squeezing or twisting the tick may cause regurgitation of infected gut contents into the skin and increase the risk of infection. Application of petroleum jelly, butter, kerosene, alcohol, fingernail polish, or a hot match will not make the tick let go and may cause the tick to inject the spirochetes into the skin.[4]

Once the tick is removed, it should be saved in a jar of alcohol for later identification. The site of the bite should be disinfected with rubbing alcohol and then watched closely for signs of erythema migrans (EM). Presumptive antibiotic treatment is probably not necessary. In endemic areas, at most 5% of detected tick bites appear to lead to symptomatic infection,[8,12–15] so it is probably better to wait for symptoms to appear before initiating treatment.

Household pets may also increase the risk of acquiring Lyme disease.[16,17] Presumably the ticks enter the house on the pet and are transferred to the owner. Pets that spend time outdoors should be fitted with tick-repellent collars and regularly brushed and inspected for ticks before they come back indoors.

Reduction of Tick Population

Biologic Control

No good biologic controls for *I. dammini* are available at present. A chalcid wasp, *Hunterellus hookeri*, parasitizes *Ixodes ricinus* and *Ixodes persulcatus* in Europe where as many as 17% of the ticks are infested in some areas.[4,5] The wasp has been introduced into *I. dammini* populations in the United States on Naushon Island, Massachusetts, and nearly 30% of the *I. dammini* there are infested, but the ticks remain extremely abundant. In other parts of eastern Massachusetts, the rate of infestation is low (< 1%). *Ixodiphagus hirtus*, another parasite, attacks *I. persulcatus* in eastern Russia, but no attempts have been made to introduce it into other tick-infested areas to date.[5]

Chemical Control

Residual application of acaricides to small areas can control vector ticks, but it is unlikely that these chemicals will be used routinely, both because of high cost and because of environmental concerns. Three chemicals registered for the control of ticks are available for use in the yard or around the home: carbaryl, chlorpyrifos, and diazinon.[4] Fall application of two of these, carbaryl and diazinon, can temporarily reduce local populations of adult *I. dammini* for up to a year, but not the number of nymphs.[18] Spring application is necessary to reduce the number of nymphs, but spraying is less likely to succeed then because the spray must penetrate the foliage and reach the leaf litter below.[4] Granular formulations of acaricide are better suited to spring and summer use and, in one study, did reduce populations of *I. dammini* nymphs (70 to 100%) and larvae (80 to 85%) compared to untreated populations when applied in mid-June and late July.[19]

An environmentally more acceptable method of chemical control is the placement of pesticide directly into the burrows of white-footed mice.[3,20,21] Tubes containing permethrin-treated cotton batting are dispersed at 10-m intervals in mouse habitats. The cotton is harvested by the mice and taken to their burrows where it is used as nesting material, and the permethrin kills the *I. dammini* larvae and nymphs in the nest. Tests of this method have shown a substantial reduction in the number of larvae feeding on mice in treated versus untreated areas.[3,20] But the number of nymphs is not lower until the second year, and there is no change in the number of larvae feeding on other hosts. The method probably works best when a large area receives full treatment, when alternate hosts are rare or absent, and when immigration into the treated area by hosts from untreated areas is limited.[21] The tubes are now commercially available, but they probably will not be used routinely as they are expensive and must be renewed twice a year.

Enviromental Modification

Environmental modification can make the habitat unsuitable for tick hatching, egg laying, molting, and host questing.[4,5] *Ixodes* ticks are vulnerable to desiccation and require high humidity, which they find in the microclimate near the soil. Mowing vegetation, removing leaf litter, and removing brush all raise the temperature and lower the humidity close to the soil and should make the environment less suitable for tick survival as well as less attractive to their hosts. In one study, mowing woodland brush did reduce the adult tick population by 70% for a year,[22] and, in another, controlled burning reduced host-seeking adults by more than 70%, also for a year.[22]

While these methods of environmental modification, though effective, will not be acceptable in most areas, other less drastic methods will be. The homeowner can maintain a closely cut lawn, remove brush piles favored by mice, locate wood piles away from the house, keep rock walls free of vegetation, and relocate bird feeders away from the house and cease feeding entirely during the spring and summer when the juvenile ticks are active.[4,5]

Denial of Access to Host Animals

Denial of tick access to animal hosts is another preventive strategy that may be of value in special circumstances. In areas of Europe where adult *I. ricinus* feed mainly on sheep, pasture rotation has led to a sharp decrease in the number of larval ticks.[3]

In North America, the increasing prevalence and spread of Lyme disease appear to be linked to the recent resurgence in deer populations, suggesting that the tick could be controlled by reducing the number of deer. In one experiment on Great Island, Massachusetts, numbers of ticks did not change until the deer population was nearly totally eliminated, however.[23] Then the numbers of larval and nymphal *I. dammini* were decreased in each of the next three summers, but the number of questing adults increased. Moreover, deer elimination as a preventive strategy is only practical on small islands or in other geographically isolated areas, and even there it is unlikely to be a popular option.

Finally, even if these methods fail, and infection occurs anyway, neurologic involvement can still be prevented in most cases if antibiotics are prescribed promptly. Therefore, individuals at risk must be aware of the early symptoms of Lyme disease and must consult their physicians at the first sign of the illness.

References

1. Johnson RC, Kodner CL, Russell ME. Vaccination of hamsters against experimental infection with *Borrelia burgdorferi. Zentralbl Bakteriol Mikrobiol Hyg [A]* 1986;263:45–48.
2. Fikrig E, Barthold SW, Kantor FS, Flavell RA. Protection of mice against the Lyme disease agent by immunizing with recombinant osp A. *Science* 1990;250:553–556.
3. Spielman A. Prospects for suppressing transmission of Lyme disease. *Ann NY Acad Sci* 1988;539:212–220.
4. Stafford KC. Lyme disease prevention: Personal protection and prospects for tick control. *Conn Med* 1989;53:347–351.
5. Anderson JF. Preventing Lyme disease. *Rheum Dis Clin North Am* 1989;15:757–766.
6. Wilson ML, Litwin TS, Gavin TA. Microgeographic distribution of deer and of *Ixodes dammini*: Options for reducing the risk of Lyme disease. *Ann NY Acad Sci* 1988;539:437–439.
7. Schulze TL, Parkin WE, Bosler EM. Vector tick populations and Lyme disease: A summary of control strategies. *Ann NY Acad Sci* 1988;539:172–179.
8. Falco RC, Fish D. A survey of tick bites acquired in a Lyme disease endemic area in southern New York State. *Ann NY Acad Sci* 1988;539:456–457.
9. Insect repellents. *Med Lett Drugs Ther* 1989;31:45–47.
10. Schreck CE, Snoddy EL, Spielman A. Pressurized sprays of permethrin or deet on military clothing for personal protection against *Ixodes dammini* (Acari: Ixodidae). *J Med Entomol* 1986;23:396–399.
11. Piesman J, Mather TN, Sinsky RJ, Spielman A. Duration of tick attachment and *Borrelia burgdorferi* transmission. *J Clin Microbiol* 1987;25:557–558.
12. Paul H, Gerth H-J, Ackermann R. Infectiousness for humans of *Ixodes ricinus* containing *Borrelia burgdorferi. Zentralbl Bakteriol Mikrobiol Hyg [A]* 1986;263:473–476.
13. Costello CM, Steere AC, Pinkerton RE, Feder HM. A prospective study of tick bites in an endemic area for Lyme disease. *J Infect Dis* 1989;159:136–139.
14. Gerth H-J, Paul H, Sander M, Döller G. Risk of asymptomatic and symptomatic *Borrelia burgdorferi*–infection after natural exposure to *Ixodes ricinus* carrying *Borrelia burgdorferi* in south Germany. Presented at the Fourth International Conference on Lyme Borreliosis; June 18–21, 1990; Stockholm, Sweden.
15. Gerber MA, Shapiro ED, Persing DH, Feder HM, Luger SW. Risk of developing Lyme disease after a deer tick bite. Presented at the Fourth International Conference on Lyme Borreliosis; June 18–21, 1990; Stockholm, Sweden.
16. Steere AC, Broderick TF, Malawista SE. Erythema chronicum migrans and Lyme arthritis: Epidemiologic evidence for a tick vector. *Am J Epidemiol* 1978;108:312–321.
17. Lane RS, Lavoie PE. Lyme borreliosis in California: Acarological, clinical, and epidemiological studies. *Ann NY Acad Sci* 1988;539:192–203.
18. Schulze TL, McDevitt WM, Parkin WE, Shisler JK. Effectiveness of two insecticides in controlling *Ixodes dammini* (Acari: Ixodidae) following an outbreak of Lyme disease in New Jersey. *J Med Entomol* 1987;24:420–424.
19. Schulze TL, Bosler EM, Taylor GC, Daley JG, Shisler JK. Chemical control of all post-embryonic stages of the northern deer tick (*Ixodes dammini*) in various ecological associations in Northeastern USA. Presented at the Fourth International Conference on Lyme Borreliosis; June 18–21, 1990; Stockholm, Sweden.

20. Mather TM, Ribeiro JMC, Moore SI, Spielman A. Reducing transmission of Lyme disease spirochetes in a suburban setting. *Ann NY Acad Sci* 1988;539:402–403.
21. Ginsberg HS. Ecological factors influencing the efficacy of permethrin-treated cotton balls on *Ixodes dammini* at a national park site in New York, USA. Presented at the Fourth International Conference on Lyme Borreliosis; June 18–21, 1990; Stockholm, Sweden.
22. Wilson ML. Reduced abundance of adult *Ixodes dammini* (Acari: Ixodidae) following destruction of vegetation. *J Econ Entomol* 1986;79:693–696.
23. Wilson ML, Telford SR, Piesman J, Spielman A. Reduced abundance of immature *Ixodes dammini* (Acari: Ixodidae) following elimination of deer. *J Med Entomol* 1988;25:224–228.

Index

Color Plates

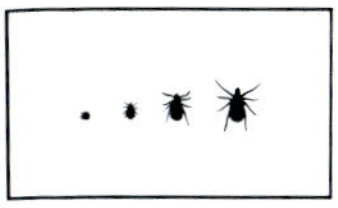

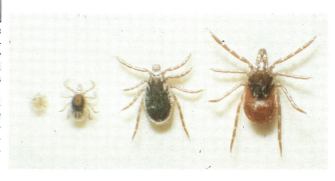

Color Plate 2–1. *Ixodes dammini*, the most important North American vector of Lyme disease, magnified approximately 10 times (from left to right: larva, nymph, adult male, and adult female). Silhouette shows actual size. (Photograph courtesy of M. Fergione, Pfizer Central Research, Groton, CT.)

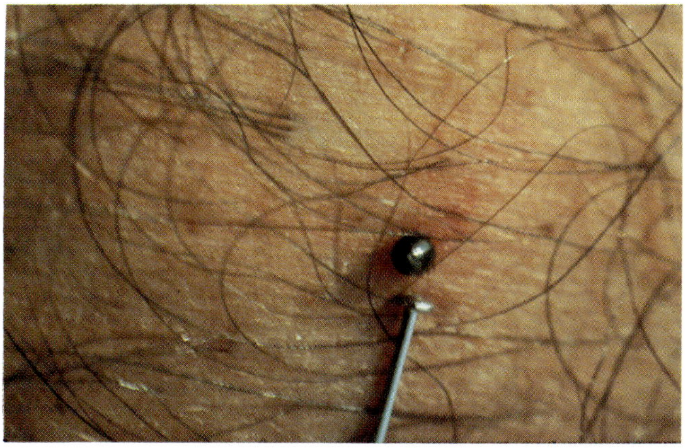

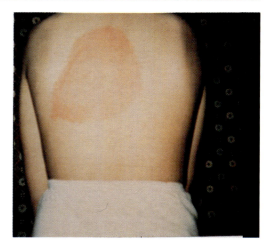

Color Plate 2–2. Nymph of *Ixodes dammini* in the act of drawing blood shown in relation to a common pin to illustrate its small size even when engorged. (Photograph courtesy of M. Fergione, Pfizer Cental Research, Groton, CT.)

Color Plate 6–1. Single large erythema migrans lesion on the upper back. (Reproduced with permission from Steere AC, Malawista SE, Hardin JA, Ruddy S, Askenase PW, Andiman WA. *Ann Intern Med* 1977; 86:685–698.)

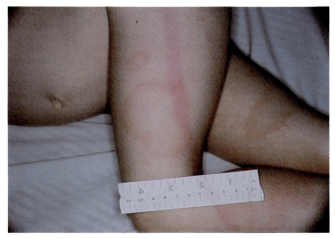

Color Plate 6–2. Multiple secondary erythema migrans on the legs. (Reproduced with permission from Steere AC, Malawista SE, Hardin JA, Ruddy S, Askenase PW, Andiman WA. *Ann Intern Med* 1977; 86:695–698.)

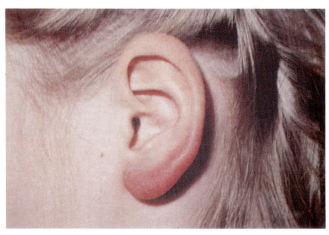

Color Plate 6–3. Borrelial lymphocytoma of 8 weeks' duration on the earlobe of a 10-year-old girl, which began 6 weeks after a tick bite. (Reproduced with permission from Weber K, Schierz G, Wilske B, Preac-Mursik V. *Yale J Biol Med* 1984;57:463–471.)

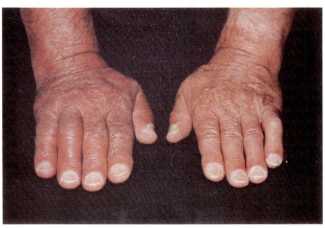

Color Plate 6–4. Acrodermatitis chronica atrophicans of 1 year's duration in a 68-year-old man. The right hand is swollen and violaceous. (Reproduced with permission from Weber K, Schierz G, Wilske B, Preac-Mursik V. *Yale J Biol Med* 1984;57:463–471.)